THE CANCER DIET COOKBOOK

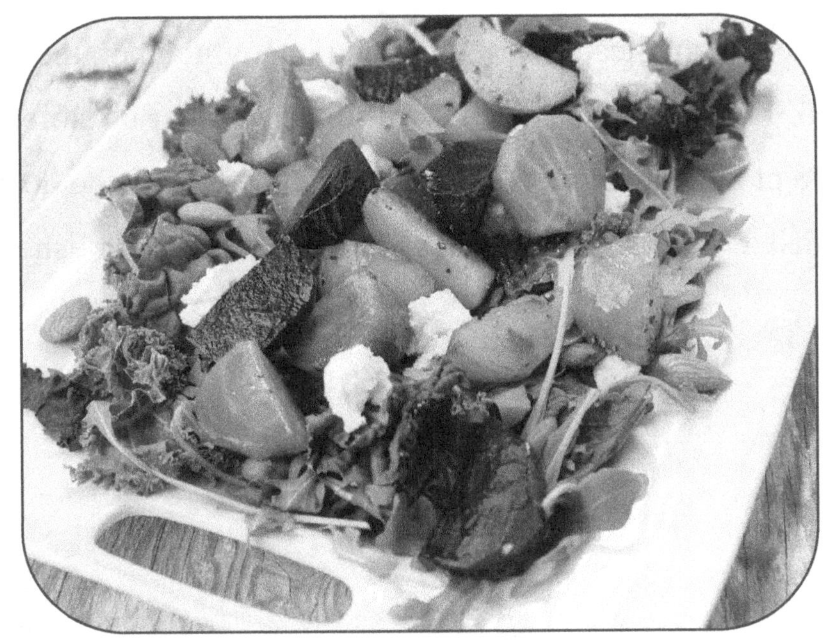

Healthy and Nutritious recipes for treating, improving, and recovery.

KERRY O. SMITH

COPYRIGHT

Copyright © by Kerry O. Smith 2024. All rights reserved.

TABLE OF CONTENTS

INTRODUCTION

As a registered dietitian, I've seen firsthand the huge impact that food choices have on our health, especially when dealing with a cancer diagnosis. Cancer treatment, while necessary in combating the disease, can frequently leave you feeling tired and dealing with side symptoms such as fatigue, nausea, and appetite problems. The good news is that nutrition may become an effective tool in your fight, allowing you to support your body's natural healing capacities and navigate treatment with greater resilience.

Imagine your body as a battlefield. Cancer interrupts the normal functioning of cells, and treatment seeks to eradicate the abnormal cells. However, this fight also impacts healthy cells, resulting in adverse consequences. This is where nutrition comes in as your secret weapon. By giving your body the correct building blocks through critical vitamins, minerals, protein, and healthy fats - it gains the strength it requires to heal, tolerate therapy, and sustain general well-being. Every bite you take is a strategic decision. Filling your plate with nutrient-rich fruits, vegetables, and whole grains provides your body with antioxidants that help combat free radicals – harmful molecules that damage healthy cells. Lean protein sources, like fish, chicken, or beans, deliver the building blocks needed to repair tissues and support a strong immune system. Healthy fats, found in nuts, seeds, and avocados, provide essential fatty acids for energy production and cell function. By consciously choosing these foods, you are actively nourishing your body and bolstering its defenses.

Of all, dealing with a cancer diagnosis may be emotionally draining, and the idea of meal planning may seem like an extra weight. But here's the key: tiny, good adjustments can have a significant impact. Begin by focusing on adding more fruits and vegetables to your everyday routine. Perhaps it's having a vibrant fruit salad for breakfast or serving roasted vegetables with your dinner. Choose lean protein sources that you prefer, and don't be afraid to try new cooking techniques like baking or grilling to preserve nutrients.

The journey does not have to be done alone. As your registered dietitian, I am here to work with you. We can collaborate to develop a personalized nutrition plan that takes into account your unique needs, taste preferences, and medication side effects. I can answer your questions, offer advice on how to manage side effects through diet, and suggest meal-planning ideas that make healthy eating easy and pleasant.

Cancer therapy is a marathon, not a sprint. Understanding the power of nutrition and adopting intelligent food choices will enable your body to fight back and recover with more vigor and energy. Remember, you are not simply a patient; you are a fighter, and proper diet is your armor.

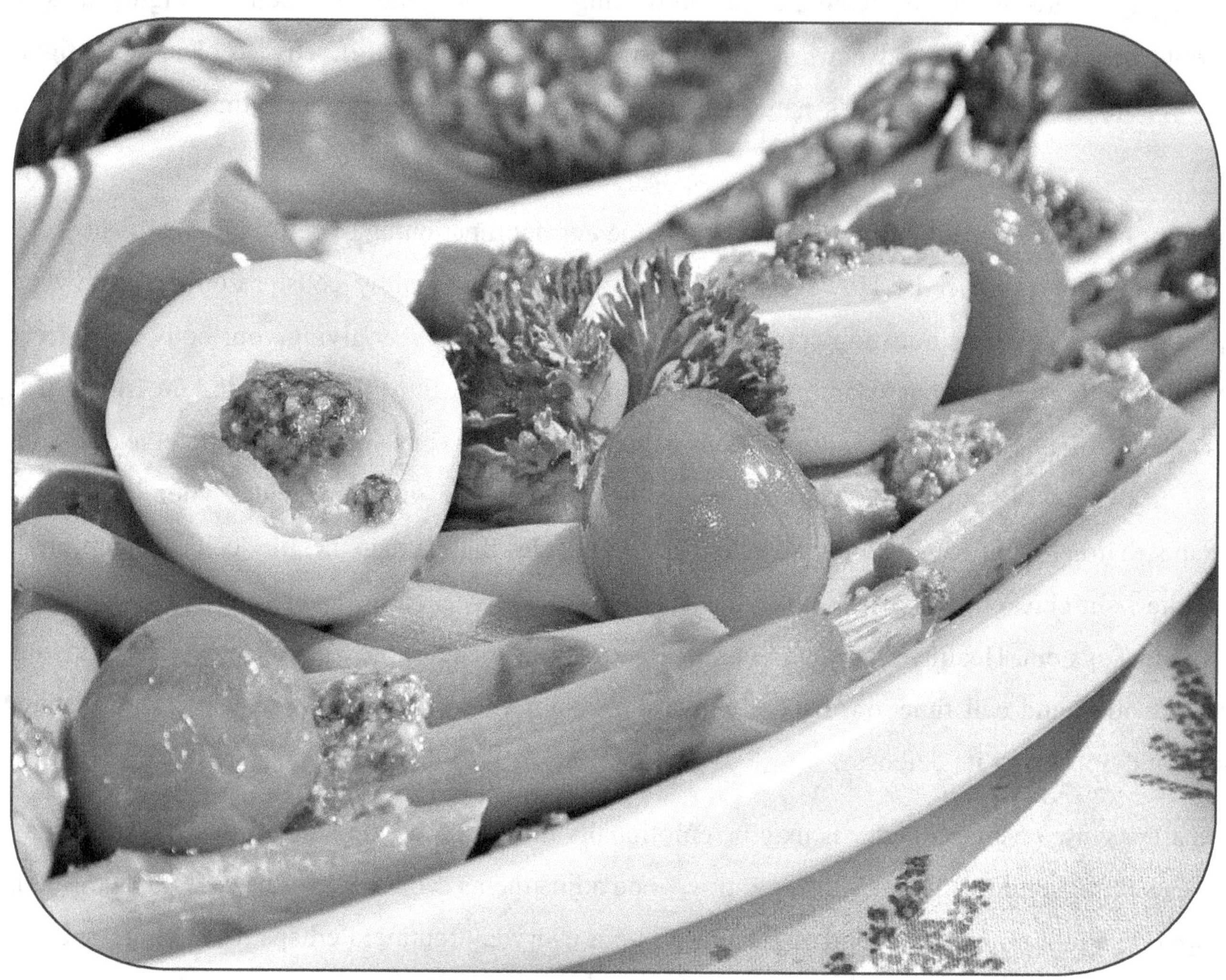

How This Cookbook Can Help You

Think of this book as your personalized toolbox, and most importantly, you'll find a vast array of delicious and easy-to-prepare recipes that cater to a variety of tastes and preferences.

<u>**Here's how this cookbook can become your indispensable buddy:**</u>

1. **Building a Cancer-Fighting Plate:** Forget restrictive diets. This book focuses on building a balanced and colorful plate that provides your body with the essential nutrients it needs to heal. We'll explore the importance of protein sources for tissue repair, the power of fruits and vegetables packed with antioxidants, and the role of healthy fats for sustained energy. Each recipe is meticulously crafted with these principles in mind, ensuring you get the right "fuel" to fight the battle.

2. **Managing Treatment Side Effects**: Cancer treatment can unfortunately come with a cocktail of unpleasant side effects. This book offers dietary strategies to help you navigate these challenges. Whether you're struggling with nausea, fatigue, or changes in taste, you'll find recipes specifically designed to be gentle on your stomach, easy to digest, and packed with flavor to entice a diminished appetite. We'll also explore helpful tips for maintaining hydration through refreshing beverages and managing mouth sores with soothing options.

3. **Convenience and Flexibility:** Let's face it, during treatment, every ounce of energy is precious. This book prioritizes your well-being by offering a variety of quick and easy recipes. We'll explore batch-cooking techniques for busy days, meal-prepping strategies to save time, and smart substitutions to accommodate dietary restrictions or personal preferences. Keep in mind, maintaining a healthy diet doesn't need to be intricate!

4. **A World of Flavorful Options:** One of the biggest concerns I hear from patients is the fear of losing the joy of food during treatment. This book combats that fear with a diverse array of

delicious recipes. From comforting soups and stews to light and refreshing salads, from protein-packed breakfasts to energizing snacks, you'll find dishes to tantalize your taste buds and keep your culinary spirit thriving. Remember, good nutrition shouldn't be bland or boring!

But perhaps the most important aspect of this cookbook is its focus on empowerment. By providing you with the knowledge and tools to make informed dietary choices, this book puts you in control of your well-being. You'll walk away feeling confident in your ability to navigate your cancer journey with strength, resilience, and a renewed appreciation for the power of good food.

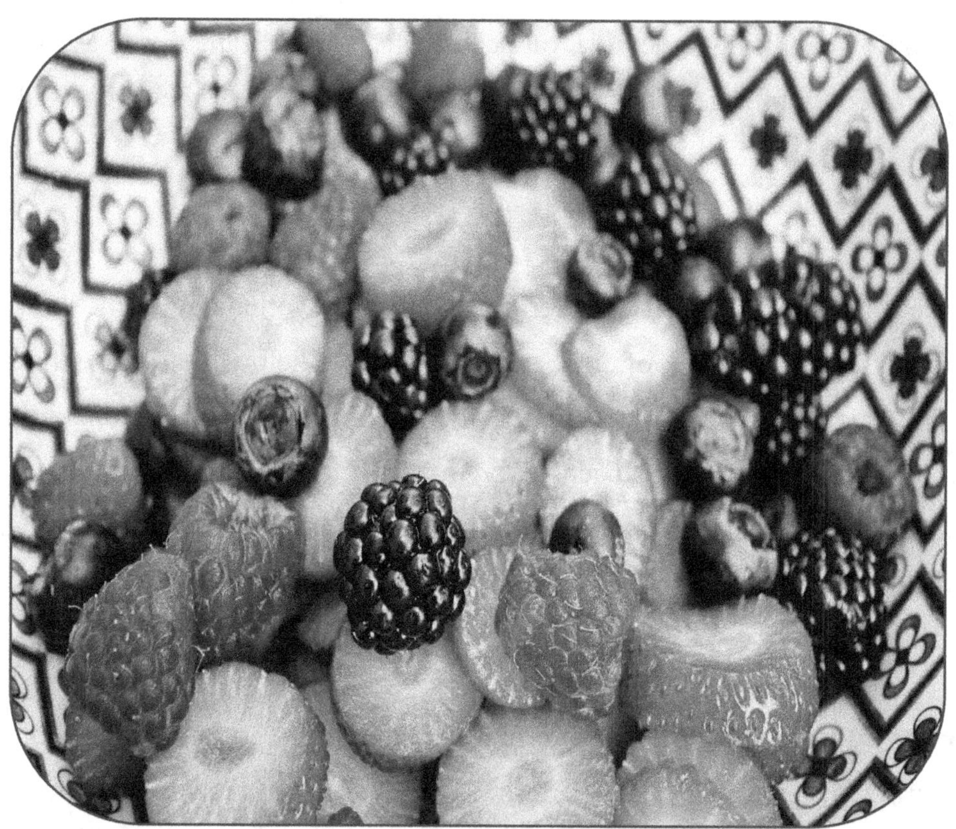

CHAPTER 1

THE IMPACT OF CANCER ON THE BODY AND NUTRITIONAL NEEDS

Understanding How Cancer Affects Metabolism

Cancer is a complicated and varied disease that affects not only cells in the body but also many metabolic systems, resulting in changes in nutritional requirements. To effectively battle cancer and promote general health, it is critical to understand the complex ways in which the disease affects metabolism and dietary requirements.

Specific sensors can detect a wide range of metabolites (mostly the three primary nutrients and their derivatives), which subsequently activate a number of signal transduction pathways and influence gene expression levels in epigenetics, a process known as **metabolite sensing**. The life body regulates metabolism, immunity, and inflammation by metabolite sensing, coordinating the host's pathophysiology to attain equilibrium with the external environment. Metabolic reprogramming in malignancies causes cancer cells to have distinct phenotypic traits than normal cells, such as cell **proliferation, migration, invasion**, and **angiogenesis.**

One of the distinguishing features of cancer metabolism is enhanced glucose absorption and use by malignant cells. The Warburg effect causes increased glycolysis, which is the breakdown of glucose to provide energy even in the presence of oxygen. As a result, people with cancer may have higher blood glucose levels and a larger need for carbohydrates to meet the energy demands of both malignant and normal cells.

Metabolic abnormalities in cancer cells create a microenvironment rich in oncometabolites that promote cancer growth, resulting in a vicious circle. Exogenous metabolites, on the other hand, have the potential to influence tumor biology. In this discussion, we explore the mechanisms by which the body senses metabolites from the three primary nutrients and their derivatives, along with how abnormalities in these processes contribute to the development of different cancers. Additionally, we delve into potential therapeutic targets that stem from signaling pathways involved in metabolite sensing, aiming to impede the progression of cancer.

Furthermore, cancer and its therapies can cause a variety of metabolic changes that affect nutritional requirements and diet tolerance. For example, chemotherapy and radiation therapy can cause nausea, vomiting, taste changes, and appetite suppression, making it difficult for patients to eat a healthy diet. Furthermore, certain malignancies, such as pancreatic cancer, might affect nutrient absorption and digestion, worsening malnutrition and weight loss.

Given these metabolic intricacies, it is critical to tailor nutrition therapies to each cancer patient's specific needs. Understanding how cancer impacts metabolism and nutritional requirements allows healthcare providers to create individualized dietary recommendations targeted at improving treatment outcomes, increasing quality of life, and promoting general well-being.

Vital Nutrients to Support Cancer Treatment and Recovery

As a registered dietitian who specializes in oncology nutrition, I realize how important nutrition is in helping people through their cancer journey. Proper nutrition not only helps manage treatment side effects and maintain overall health, but it also improves the body's ability to fight cancer and recover efficiently. In this section, I will go over some essential nutrients that are especially good for people undergoing cancer treatment and rehabilitation.

1. **Protein:**

Protein is often referred to as the building block of life, and its importance cannot be overstated, especially for cancer patients. Adequate protein intake is essential for supporting immune function, preserving muscle mass, and promoting tissue repair and healing. During cancer treatment, the body's protein needs may increase due to factors such as tissue damage, metabolic alterations, and the body's response to stress. Including high-quality protein sources in each meal and snack, such as lean meats, poultry, fish, eggs, dairy products, legumes, and tofu, can help meet these increased requirements and support optimal recovery.

2. **Omega-3 fatty acids:**

Omega-3 fatty acids, found primarily in fatty fish, flaxseeds, chia seeds, walnuts, and hemp seeds, possess anti-inflammatory properties that can be particularly beneficial for individuals with cancer. Chronic inflammation is a common feature of cancer and its treatment, contributing to symptoms such as pain, fatigue, and decreased appetite. Consuming foods rich in omega-3 fatty acids may help mitigate inflammation, improve treatment tolerance, and enhance overall well-being. Additionally, omega-3 fatty acids have been associated with reduced cancer-related cachexia, a debilitating condition characterized by severe weight loss and muscle wasting.

3. Antioxidants:

Antioxidants are compounds that help neutralize harmful free radicals in the body, thereby protecting cells from oxidative damage. Cancer treatments such as chemotherapy and radiation therapy can generate oxidative stress, leading to tissue damage and inflammation. Including antioxidant-rich foods in the diet, such as fruits, vegetables, nuts, seeds, and whole grains, can help counteract this oxidative stress and support cellular health. Colorful fruits and vegetables, in particular, are abundant sources of vitamins, minerals, and phytochemicals with potent antioxidant properties.

4. Vitamin D:

Vitamin D plays a crucial role in immune function, bone health, and inflammation regulation, making it a valuable nutrient for individuals undergoing cancer treatment. Low levels of vitamin D have been associated with increased cancer risk, disease progression, and treatment-related complications. Sun exposure and dietary sources such as fatty fish, fortified dairy products, and fortified cereals can help maintain adequate vitamin D levels. However, supplementation may be necessary for individuals with insufficient sun exposure or impaired vitamin D absorption.

5. Fluids and hydration:

Proper hydration is essential for supporting numerous physiological functions, including nutrient transport, toxin elimination, and tissue hydration. Cancer treatments such as chemotherapy and radiation therapy can increase the risk of dehydration due to side effects such as nausea, vomiting, diarrhea, and mucositis. Encouraging adequate fluid intake, preferably from water, herbal teas, broths, and hydrating foods like fruits and vegetables, can help prevent dehydration and support overall wellness.

Foods to Embrace for Optimal Health

1. Fruits and Vegetables

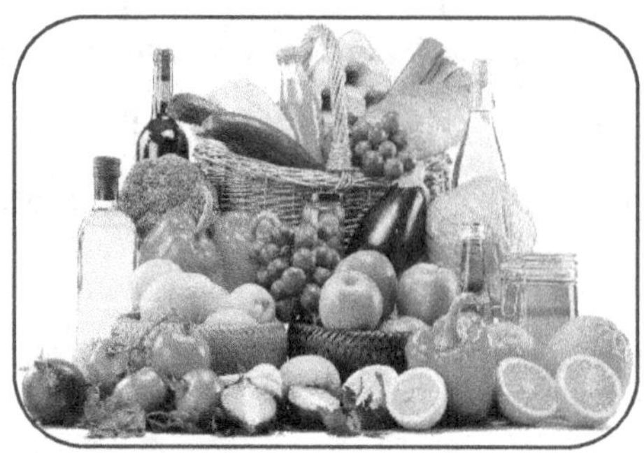

Rich in vitamins, minerals, antioxidants, and phytochemicals, fruits and vegetables are essential components of a cancer-fighting diet. These vibrant foods help combat oxidative stress, reduce inflammation, and support immune function. Aim to include a rainbow of colors on your plate, such as leafy greens, berries, citrus fruits, carrots, bell peppers, and cruciferous vegetables like broccoli and Brussels sprouts.

2. Whole Grains

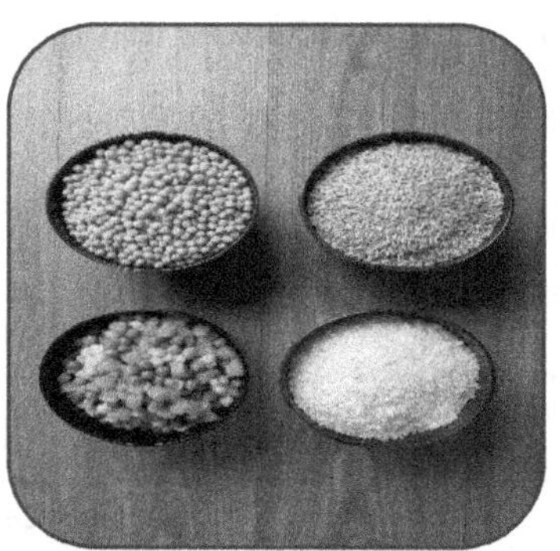

Whole grains like brown rice, quinoa, and whole-wheat bread are your body's slow-burning energy source. Unlike refined grains that leave you feeling sluggish, whole grains provide sustained energy thanks to their complex carbohydrates and fiber content. Fiber also keeps you feeling fuller for longer, which can be helpful if you're struggling with nausea or a decreased appetite. Plus, whole grains are packed with B vitamins essential for energy production and cell health.

3. Lean Protein

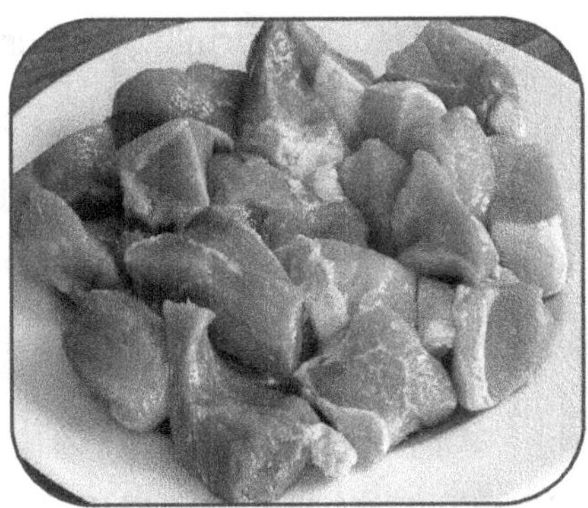

Protein is the building block of life, and during cancer treatment, your body needs ample amounts to repair tissues damaged by the disease and its treatment. Lean protein sources like fish, chicken, beans, and lentils are your MVPs. Fish, especially fatty fish like salmon, are rich in omega-3 fatty acids, which have been shown to have anti-inflammatory properties. Beans and lentils are fantastic options for vegetarians and vegans, providing complete protein with a healthy dose of fiber.

4. Healthy Fats

Don't let the "bad fat" misconception fool you. Healthy fats from sources like avocado, nuts, and olive oil are crucial for your health. These fats provide essential fatty acids that your body needs for energy production and cell function. They also help your body absorb fat-soluble vitamins like A, D, E, and K. Of course, moderation is key, so opt for a drizzle of olive oil instead of a drench, and enjoy a handful of nuts instead of a whole bag.

5. Hydrating fluids:

Staying hydrated is essential for maintaining overall health and supporting various bodily functions, especially during cancer treatment. Aim to drink plenty of fluids throughout the day, including water, herbal teas, broths, and freshly squeezed juices. Hydrating foods like fruits, vegetables, and soups also contribute to your daily fluid intake.

Foods to Limit or Avoid During Treatment

> **Added Sugars and Refined Carbohydrates:** Think of sugary drinks, processed pastries, and white bread as empty calories. They offer little to no nutritional value and can cause blood sugar spikes, which can be especially detrimental if you're managing diabetes alongside cancer. These refined carbohydrates also lack the fiber found in whole grains, leaving you feeling hungry sooner. Opt for natural sweeteners like fruits or a sprinkle of honey, and choose whole grain options over their refined counterparts.

> **Processed Meats and Unhealthy Fats:** Processed meats like hot dogs, sausages, and deli meats are often high in sodium and nitrates, which have been linked to an increased risk of certain cancers. Unhealthy fats, found in fried foods and processed snacks, can contribute to inflammation in the body. Instead, focus on lean protein sources like grilled chicken or fish, and choose healthy fats from sources like avocado, nuts, and olive oil.

> **Foods That May Interfere with Treatment:** While some foods are generally healthy, during cancer treatment, they might interact with certain medications. For instance, grapefruit can interfere with some chemotherapy drugs. It's crucial to discuss any potential food-drug interactions with your doctor or registered dietitian.

> **Beware of Misinformation:** The internet can be a treasure trove of information, but it's also rife with myths and misconceptions. Let's dispel a common one: there's no magic bullet food that "cures" cancer. A balanced diet rich in fruits, vegetables, and whole grains is the key to providing your body with the nutrients it needs to fight back.

> **Focus on What You Can Control:** Cancer treatment can be overwhelming, and sometimes, the thought of drastically changing your diet can feel like an additional burden. Here's the good news: even small changes can make a big difference. Focus on what you can control. Start by limiting processed foods and sugary drinks. Add a side of steamed vegetables to your meals. Swap white bread for whole-wheat. These seemingly small steps, when implemented consistently, contribute significantly to your overall well-being.

Taking Control of your Symptoms Through Diet

Cancer treatment, while necessary in the fight against the disease, can often feel like a double-edged sword. While it targets cancer cells, it may cause a number of unpleasant side effects. Do not be afraid, warrior! By strategically using food, you can manage some of these adverse effects and navigate treatment more comfortably.

- **Nausea and Vomiting**

One of the most common side effects is nausea and vomiting. The thought of food can be repulsive, but skipping meals can actually worsen the problem. The key is to find small, frequent meals that sit well with your stomach. Ginger, a natural anti-nausea fighter, can be your BFF. Try sipping on ginger tea or nibbling on crystallized ginger candies. Bland, easily digestible options like crackers, toast, or plain rice might be more appealing than heavy or greasy foods. Cold or room-temperature foods are often easier on the stomach than hot meals. Remember, listen to your body. If something feels off, avoid pushing it. There will be other opportunities to nourish yourself.

- **Fatigue**

Fatigue can feel like a heavy cloak draped over you, sapping your energy for even the simplest tasks. The good news is that dietary choices can help combat this energy drain. Direct your attention to consuming complex carbohydrates like whole grains, fruits, and vegetables. These provide sustained energy as your body slowly breaks them down, unlike sugary snacks that offer a quick burst followed by a crash. Staying hydrated is also crucial. Aim for water throughout the day, and consider incorporating hydrating fruits and vegetables like watermelon or cucumber. Small, frequent meals will keep your blood sugar levels stable, preventing those energy dips.

- **Loss of Appetite**

A diminished appetite can make it challenging to get the nutrients you need. The trick is to focus on smaller, more frequent meals packed with flavor. Experiment with different spices and herbs to add zip to your dishes. Small, nutrient-dense snacks like nuts, seeds, or yogurt with fruit can be a great way to sneak in extra calories and nutrients throughout the day. Soups and smoothies are also excellent options. They're easy to digest and can be packed with protein and vitamins. Don't be afraid to get creative! Presentation can also play a role. Colorful, visually appealing meals might be more enticing than a bland plate of food.

- **Mouth Sores and Difficulty Swallowing**

Mouth sores and difficulty swallowing can make the simple act of eating a painful experience. The key is to choose soft, smooth foods that are easy to chew and swallow. Mashed potatoes, applesauce, yogurt, and scrambled eggs are great options. Soups are a lifesaver – they're hydrating, provide essential nutrients, and are easy to swallow. Cold or room-temperature foods might be more soothing than hot or spicy dishes. Remember, it's okay to prioritize pureed or blended foods until your mouth heals. Your body still needs the nutrients, and there's no shame in making mealtime a little easier on yourself.

HAPPY DIETING!!!

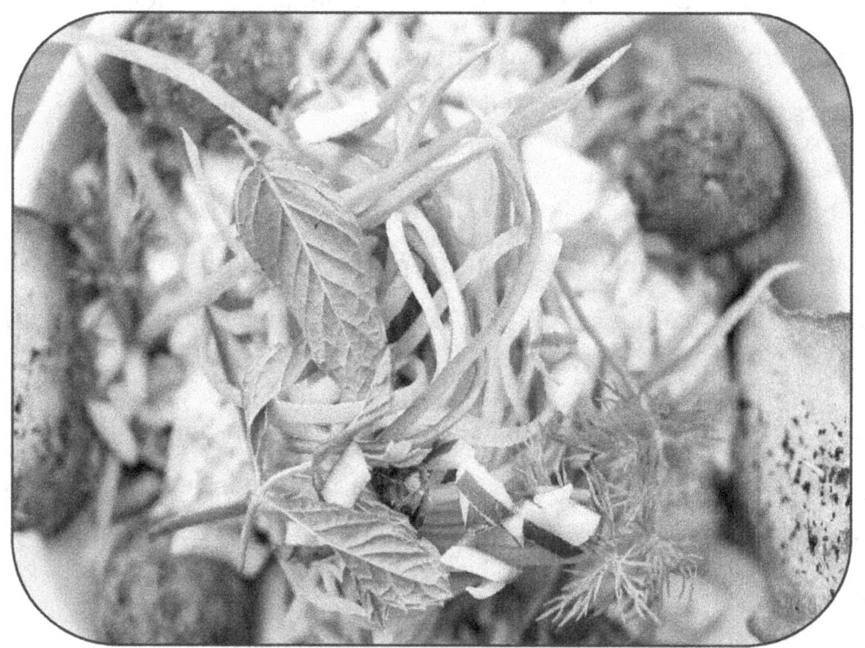

CHAPTER 2

BREAKFAST

Cranberry Flax Pumpkin Bread

Serving size: 1/12th of the loaf, PREP Time: 15-20 minutes, Baking Time: 45 to 55 minutes, Total time: 1 hour and 15 minutes.

Ingredients

- Canola oil spray
- 1/2 cup whole-wheat pastry flour
- 1/2 cup unbleached all-purpose flour
- 1/2 cup ground flaxseed
- 2/3 cup packed light brown sugar
- 1 tsp. baking soda
- 1/2 tsp. salt
- 2 large eggs
- 1 cup canned pumpkin
- 1/4 cup canola oil
- 1/2 cup unsweetened applesauce
- 1/4 cup 100 percent apple juice
- 1/2 tsp. ground cinnamon
- 1/2 tsp. ground ginger
- 1/4 tsp. ground nutmeg
- 1 cup dried cranberries

Directions

1. Preheat the oven to 350 degrees F. Lightly coat an 8 x 4-inch loaf pan with canola oil spray and set aside.

2. In a sizable bowl, mix together whole-wheat pastry flour, all-purpose flour, flaxseed, sugar, baking soda, and salt, then set it aside. In a medium bowl, lightly beat eggs. Blend together pumpkin, canola oil, applesauce, apple juice, cinnamon, ginger, and nutmeg using a whisk, Stir in dried cranberries. Add wet ingredients to dry ingredients, mixing until all dry ingredients are incorporated into the batter. Do not beat or overmix. Pour batter into the prepared pan.

3. Bake for 50-60 minutes, until a wooden toothpick inserted into the center comes out clean. Allow the bread to cool in a pan on a wire rack for 10 minutes. Then, remove it from the pan and continue cooling on the rack.

Chard with Feta and Egg Breakfast Toast

Servings: 1 person, PREP Time: 10 minutes, Cook Time: 10 minutes

Ingredients:

- 1 tablespoon olive oil
- 2 large chard leaves, chopped
- 1/4 cup crumbled feta cheese
- 1 hard-boiled egg, thinly sliced
- 1 slice whole-wheat toast
- Salt and freshly ground black pepper to taste

Direction

1. Toast bread.
2. Sauté chard in olive oil until soft and reduced by about ¾ in size.
3. Spread it atop your toast, sprinkle with feta, and top with a hard-boiled egg.
4. you can add salt and pepper if you want if it to taste.

Nutritional Information (per serving):

Calories: 280

Fat: 14g

Saturated Fat: 4g

Cholesterol: 180mg

Sodium: 320mg (depending on the feta cheese)

Carbohydrates: 22g

Fiber: 4g

Sugar: 3g

Protein: 16g

Homemade Granola with Berries

Serving size: 1/2 cup, Prep Time: 10 minutes, Cook Time: 25 minutes

Ingredients:

- 2 cups old-fashioned rolled oats (use certified gluten-free oats for gluten-free granola)
- ¼ cup raw nuts and/or seeds (almonds, walnuts, sunflower seeds, chia seeds – choose your favorites!)
- ¼ teaspoon ground cinnamon
- ¼ teaspoon ground ginger (optional, for a touch of anti-inflammatory goodness)
- Pinch of fine-grain sea salt
- ¼ cup melted coconut oil (or olive oil)
- ¼ cup honey or maple syrup
- ½ cup dried cranberries (or other dried fruits you enjoy)

Directions:

1. Start by pre-heating your oven down to about 350 degrees Fahrenheit (175 degrees Celsius). Line a baking sheet with parchment paper.
2. In a large bowl, combine the rolled oats, nuts/seeds, cinnamon, ginger (if using), and salt. Stir well.
3. In a separate bowl, whisk together the melted coconut oil and honey/maple syrup. Pour the liquid ingredients into the dry ingredients and stir until they are evenly coated.
4. Spread the granola mixture onto the prepared baking sheet, forming an even layer. Use a spatula to gently press down on the granola for better clumping (optional).

5. Bake the granola for 20-25 minutes, stirring halfway through. The granola should be lightly golden brown and toasted.

6. Remove the pan from the oven and let the granola cool completely on the baking sheet.

7. Once cool, stir in the dried cranberries and break up any large clumps of granola.

Nutritional Information (per 1/2 cup serving):

Calories: 280

Fat: 12g

Saturated Fat: 6g

Carbohydrates: 32g

Fiber: 4g

Sugar: 12g

Protein: 5g

Power-Packed Hot Cereal with Berries

Serving size: 1 cup, Prep Time: 5 minutes, Cook Time: 10 minutes

Ingredients:

- ½ cup rolled oats (use certified gluten-free oats for a gluten-free version)
- ½ cup unsweetened plant-based milk (almond milk, soy milk, etc.)
- ¼ cup water
- 1 scoop protein powder (unflavored or vanilla works well)
- ½ cup of fresh or frozen berries such as blueberries, raspberries, or strawberries.
- Pinch of ground cinnamon
- Optional toppings: Sliced almonds, chia seeds, chopped banana

Directions:

1. In a saucepan, combine the rolled oats, plant-based milk, water, and protein powder.

2. Heat the mixture over medium heat, stirring occasionally, until it reaches a desired consistency (creamy or slightly thicker).

3. Remove from heat and stir in the berries and cinnamon.

4. Pour the hot cereal into a bowl and top with your favorite options like sliced almonds, chia seeds, or chopped banana.

Nutritional Information (per 1 cup serving, without toppings):

Calories: 300

Fat: 5g

Saturated Fat: 1g

Carbohydrates: 40g

Fiber: 5g

Sugar: (varies depending on berries used)

Protein: 20g (based on a 20g scoop of protein powder)

Berry Baked Oatmeal

Serving size: 1 small dish, Prep Time: 10 minutes, Cook Time: 35-40 minutes

Ingredients:

- ½ cup mashed banana (about ½ of a ripe banana)
- ½ cup rolled oats (use certified gluten-free oats for a gluten-free version)
- ¼ cup unsweetened plant-based milk
- 1 scoop unflavored protein powder
- ¼ teaspoon ground cinnamon
- Pinch of ground ginger (optional)
- ¼ cup fresh or frozen berries
- ¼ cup chopped walnuts or pecans (optional)

Directions:

1. Heat your oven to 350 degrees Fahrenheit (175 degrees Celsius) before starting. Lightly grease a small baking dish (ramekin or small baking pan).
2. In a large bowl, mash the banana with a fork until mostly smooth. Stir in the rolled oats, plant-based milk, protein powder, cinnamon, and ginger (if using).
3. Fold in the berries and chopped nuts (if using).
4. Transfer the oatmeal mixture into the baking dish that has been prepared.
5. Bake for 35-40 minutes, or until the oatmeal is set and the top is slightly golden brown.
6. Let the oatmeal cool slightly before enjoying it.

Nutritional Information (per 1 small dish, without nuts):

Calories: 250

Fat: 5g

Saturated Fat: 1g

Carbohydrates: 35g

Fiber: 4g

Sugar: (varies depending on berries used)

Protein: 15g (based on a 20g scoop of protein powder)

Healthy Whole-Grain Pancakes

Serving size: 2 pancakes, Prep Time: 10 minutes, Cook Time: 10 minutes

Ingredients:

- ½ cup whole wheat flour
- ½ teaspoon baking powder
- ¼ teaspoon baking soda
- ¼ teaspoon ground cinnamon
- Pinch of salt

- 1 large egg
- ½ cup unsweetened plant-based milk (almond milk, soy milk, etc.)
- 1 tablespoon of coconut oil (or olive oil) that has been melted.
- ¼ cup fresh or frozen blueberries (optional)

Directions:

1. In a medium bowl, whisk together the whole wheat flour, baking powder, baking soda, cinnamon, and salt.
2. In a separate bowl, whisk together the egg and plant-based milk. Mix in the melted coconut oil until thoroughly combined.
3. Combine the wet ingredients with the dry ones and stir until just incorporated. Don't overmix! A few lumps are okay.
4. Gently fold in the blueberries, if using.
5. Warm a lightly greased non-stick skillet over medium heat.
6. Pour ¼ cup of batter per pancake onto the skillet. Cook for 2-3 minutes, or until bubbles appear on the surface.
7. Flip the pancakes and cook for an additional 1-2 minutes or until golden brown on both sides.
8. Serve warm with your favorite toppings like fresh fruit, a drizzle of maple syrup, or a sprinkle of chopped nuts.

Nutritional Information (per 2 pancakes, without toppings):

Calories: 250

Fat: 7g

Saturated Fat: 3g

Carbohydrates: 35g

Fiber: 4g

Sugar: (trace amounts)

Protein: 8g

P a g e

Blueberry Flax Muffins

Serving size: 1 muffin, Prep Time: 10 minutes, Cook Time: 20-25 minutes

Ingredients:

- ½ cup whole wheat flour
- 1 tablespoon ground flaxseed meal
- ½ teaspoon baking powder
- ¼ teaspoon baking soda
- ¼ teaspoon ground cinnamon
- Pinch of salt
- 1 large egg, beaten
- ¼ cup unsweetened applesauce
- ¼ cup unsweetened plant-based milk
- 1 tablespoon of coconut oil (or olive oil) that has been melted.
- ¼ cup fresh or frozen blueberries

Directions:

1. Before you start, preheat your oven to 375 degrees Fahrenheit (190 degrees Celsius). Line a muffin tin with paper liners.
2. In a medium bowl, whisk together the whole wheat flour, flaxseed meal, baking powder, baking soda, cinnamon, and salt.
3. In a separate bowl, whisk together the beaten egg, applesauce, plant-based milk, and melted coconut oil.
4. Combine the liquid ingredients with the dry ingredients and stir until just blended. Carefully incorporate the blueberries.
5. Evenly distribute the batter among the muffin cups that have been prepared.
6. Bake for 20-25 minutes, or until a toothpick inserted into the center emerges clean.
7. Let the muffins cool slightly in the pan before removing them to a wire rack to cool completely.

Nutritional Information (per 1 muffin):

Calories: 220

Fat: 7g

Saturated Fat: 2g

Carbohydrates: 30g

Fiber: 4g

Sugar: (natural sugars from fruit)

Protein: 5g

Sweet Potato Porridge

Serving size: 1 cup, Prep Time: 5 minutes, Cook Time: 15-20 minutes

Ingredients:

- ½ cup diced sweet potato
- ½ cup unsweetened plant-based milk
- ¼ cup water
- 1 tablespoon rolled oats (use certified gluten-free oats for a gluten-free version)
- ¼ teaspoon ground cinnamon
- Pinch of ground ginger (optional)
- Optional toppings: Sliced almonds, chopped banana, a drizzle of honey

Directions:

1. In a small saucepan, combine the diced sweet potato, plant-based milk, water, rolled oats, cinnamon, and ginger (if using).
2. Heat the mixture until it reaches a boil on medium heat. Reduce heat to low and simmer for 15-20 minutes, or until the sweet potato is tender and the oats are cooked through. Stir occasionally to prevent sticking.
3. Remove the pan from the heat. Using an immersion blender or a regular blender, puree the mixture until it reaches a desired consistency. You can leave it slightly chunky or blend it completely smooth.

4. Pour the porridge into a bowl and top with your favorite options like sliced almonds, chopped banana, or a drizzle of honey.

Nutritional Information (per 1 cup serving):

Calories: 200

Fat: 3g

Saturated Fat: 1g

Carbohydrates: 35g

Fiber: 4g

Sugar: (natural sugars from sweet potato)

Protein: 2g (depending on the plant-based milk used)

Veggie Omelet

Serving size: 1 omelet, Prep Time: 5 minutes, Cook Time: 10 minutes

Ingredients:

- 2 large eggs
- 1 tablespoon unsweetened plant-based milk (optional, for a creamier omelet)
- ¼ teaspoon dried oregano
- Pinch of salt and black pepper
- ¼ cup chopped vegetables (spinach, mushrooms, bell peppers, onions – choose your favorites!)
- 1 tablespoon shredded cheese (optional)
- 1 tablespoon chopped fresh herbs (optional, parsley, chives)

Directions:

1. In a small bowl, whisk together the eggs, plant-based milk (if using), oregano, salt, and pepper.
2. Heat a non-stick skillet over medium heat. Spray the pan with non-stick cooking spray or coat it with a thin layer of oil.

3. Pour the beaten eggs into the skillet and swirl them around to cover the surface evenly.

4. As the omelet begins to set, add the chopped vegetables to one-half of the omelet.

5. (Optional) Sprinkle the shredded cheese over the vegetables if using.

6. Once the omelet is mostly set, use a spatula to fold the other half over the vegetables and cheese.

7. Cook for an additional minute or two, or until the cheese is melted and the omelet is cooked through.

8. Slide the omelet onto a plate and garnish with chopped fresh herbs (if using).

Nutritional Information (per 1 omelet, without cheese):

Calories: 200

Fat: 10g

Saturated Fat: 2g (depending on the cooking oil used)

Carbohydrates: 2g

Fiber: 1g

Sugar: (trace amounts)

Protein: 12g

Egg and Veggie Sandwich

(Serving size: 1 sandwich, Prep Time: 5 minutes, Cook Time: Depending on the cooking method for the egg (fried, scrambled, etc.)

Ingredients:

- 2 slices whole-wheat bread, toasted
- 1 large egg, cooked to your preference (fried, scrambled, etc.)
- ¼ cup chopped vegetables (spinach, tomatoes, avocado, cucumber – choose your favorites!)
- 1 tablespoon low-fat mayonnaise or mashed avocado (for spread)
- Salt and pepper to taste (optional)

Directions:

1. Toast the whole-wheat bread slices to your desired level of doneness.
2. Spread a thin layer of mayonnaise or mashed avocado on one slice of toast.
3. Layer the cooked egg on top of the spread.
4. Add your chosen chopped vegetables.
5. Season with salt and pepper to taste (optional).
6. Place the remaining slice of toasted bread on top and savor the dish!

Nutritional Information (per sandwich, with fried egg and mayonnaise):

Calories: 350

Fat: 18g

Saturated Fat: 4g (depending on the mayonnaise used)

Carbohydrates: 30g

Fiber: 4g (depending on bread)

Sugar: (trace amounts)

Protein: 15g

Sausage and Roasted Veggie Hash

Serving size: 1 serving, Prep Time: 10 minutes, Cook Time: 30-35 minutes

Ingredients:

- ½ cup chopped vegetables (bell peppers, onions, potatoes, sweet potatoes – choose your favorites!)
- 1 tablespoon olive oil
- ¼ teaspoon dried thyme
- Pinch of salt and black pepper
- 1 turkey or chicken sausage link (or plant-based sausage)
- 1 large egg, cooked to your preference (optional)

Directions:

1. Make sure to Preheat your oven to 400 degrees Fahrenheit (200 degrees Celsius).
2. Toss the chopped vegetables with olive oil, thyme, salt, and pepper.
3. Arrange the vegetables evenly on a baking sheet, making sure they form a single layer.
4. Roast the vegetables for 20-25 minutes or until tender and slightly browned.
5. While the vegetables are roasting, cook the sausage link according to package instructions.
6. In the last few minutes of roasting the vegetables, you can optionally add the sausage link to the baking sheet and cook it alongside the vegetables until heated through.
7. Once the vegetables and sausage are cooked, transfer them to a plate.
8. If you'd like a heartier breakfast, cook your egg (fried, scrambled, poached) to your preference.
9. Serve the roasted veggie hash with the cooked sausage link and the optional fried/scrambled/poached egg on top.

Nutritional Information (per serving, with turkey sausage and fried egg):

Calories: 400

Fat: 20g

Saturated Fat: 5g (depending on the sausage used)

Carbohydrates: 30g

Fiber: 5g (depending on vegetables used)

Sugar: (natural sugars from vegetables)

Protein: 20g (based on turkey sausage and egg)

CHAPTER 3

WHOLESOME SOUPS AND SALADS

Lentil Vegetable Soup

Serving Size: Approximately 1 1/2 cups, Prep Time: 15 minutes, Cooking Time: 30 minutes, Total Time: 45 minutes

Ingredients:

- 1 cup dried lentils, rinsed and drained
- 4 cups low-sodium vegetable broth
- 1 onion, diced
- 2 carrots, peeled and diced
- 2 celery stalks, diced
- 2 cloves garlic, minced
- 1 teaspoon ground cumin
- 1/2 teaspoon dried thyme
- 1/2 teaspoon paprika
- Salt and pepper to taste
- 2 cups chopped kale or spinach
- 1 tablespoon lemon juice
- Fresh parsley for garnish (optional)

Directions:

1. In a large pot, combine the lentils, vegetable broth, onion, carrots, celery, garlic, cumin, thyme, paprika, salt, and pepper. Heat until boiling on medium-high heat.
2. Reduce the heat to low, cover, and simmer for 20-25 minutes, or until the lentils and vegetables are tender.
3. Stir in the chopped kale or spinach and lemon juice. Continue cooking for another 5 minutes, until the greens have become limp.

4. Taste and adjust seasoning as needed.

5. Serve warm, optionally topped with fresh parsley if preferred.

Nutritional Information (per serving):

Calories: Approximately 200 kcal

Total Fat: Around 1-2 grams

Sodium: Approximately 400-500 milligrams

Total Carbohydrates: Approximately 35-40 grams

Dietary Fiber: Approximately 12-15 grams

Sugars: Approximately 6-8 grams

Protein: Around 12-15 grams

Quinoa Salad with Roasted Vegetables

Serving Size: Approximately 1 cup, Prep Time: 20 minutes, Cooking Time: 25 minutes, Total Time: 45 minutes

Ingredients:

- 1 cup quinoa, rinsed
- 2 cups low-sodium vegetable broth or water
- 2 cups assorted vegetables (like bell peppers, courgettes, cherry tomatoes, and red onion), diced
- 2 tablespoons olive oil
- Salt and pepper to taste
- 1/4 cup freshly chopped herbs (like parsley, basil, or cilantro)
- 2 tablespoons lemon juice
- Optional: crumbled feta cheese or toasted nuts/seeds for garnish

Directions:

1. Preheat the oven to 400°F (200°C). Place the chopped vegetables on a baking sheet, drizzle with olive oil, and season with salt and pepper. Roast in the oven for 20-25 minutes, or until tender and lightly browned.

2. Meanwhile, wash the quinoa thoroughly with cold water. In a pot, mix together the quinoa and vegetable broth or water. Bring to a boil, then lower the heat, cover, and let simmer for 15-20 minutes, or until the quinoa is fully cooked and the liquid has been absorbed. Take it off the heat and let it cool for a short while.

3. In a spacious bowl, mix together the prepared quinoa and the roasted vegetables. Add chopped herbs and lemon juice, and toss to combine. Taste and adjust seasoning as needed.

4. Serve the quinoa salad warm or at room temperature, garnished with crumbled feta cheese or toasted nuts/seeds if desired.

Nutritional Information (per serving):

Calories: Approximately 250 kcal

Total Fat: Around 10-12 grams

Sodium: Approximately 200-300 milligrams

Total Carbohydrates: Approximately 35-40 grams

Dietary Fiber: Approximately 5-7 grams

Sugars: Approximately 3-5 grams

Protein: Around 8-10 grams

Kale and White Bean Soup

Serving Size: Approximately 1 1/2 cups, Prep Time: 15 minutes, Cooking Time: 25 minutes, Total Time: 40 minutes

Ingredients:

- 1 tablespoon olive oil

- 1 onion, diced

- 2 cloves garlic, minced

- 2 carrots, peeled and diced

- 2 celery stalks, diced

- 4 cups low-sodium vegetable broth

- 1 can (15 ounces) of white beans, drained and washed

- 1 bunch of kale, with stems taken out and leaves diced

- 1 teaspoon dried thyme

- Salt and pepper to taste

- 2 tablespoons lemon juice

- Grated Parmesan cheese for garnish (optional)

Directions:

1. In a very big pot, warm olive oil over medium heat. Mix in the onion and garlic, cooking until they become soft and fragrant, typically around 3 to 4 minutes. Next, add the carrots and celery, and continue cooking for another 3-4 minutes. until slightly softened.

2. Add the vegetable broth and bring it to a gentle simmer. Add the white beans, kale, and dried thyme.

3. Let it simmer for 15-20 minutes, until the vegetables become soft

4. Season the soup with salt, pepper, and lemon juice to taste. Serve it hot, then garnished with grated Parmesan cheese if you want.

Nutritional Information (per serving):

Calories: Approximately 180-200 kcal

Total Fat: Around 3-4 grams

Sodium: Approximately 400-500 milligrams

Total Carbohydrates: Approximately 30-35 grams

Dietary Fiber: Approximately 8-10 grams

Sugars: Approximately 4-6 grams

Protein: Around 8-10 grams

Butternut Squash Soup

Serving Size: Approximately 1 1/2 cups, Prep Time: 15 minutes, Cooking Time: 40 minutes, Total Time: 55 minutes

Ingredients:

- 1 average-sized butternut squash, peeled, deseeded, and cut into cubes.
- 1 onion, chopped
- 2 carrots, peeled and chopped
- 2 celery stalks, chopped
- 2 cloves garlic, minced
- 4 cups low-sodium vegetable broth
- 1 teaspoon ground cinnamon
- 1/2 teaspoon ground nutmeg
- Salt and pepper to taste
- 1 tablespoon olive oil
- Optional: Greek yogurt or coconut cream for garnish

Directions:

1. In a very big pot, heat the olive oil over medium heat. Add the onion, carrots, celery, and garlic, and sauté until softened, about 5 minutes.
2. Add the butternut squash cubes, vegetable broth, cinnamon, and nutmeg to the pot. Bring to a boil, then reduce the heat to low and simmer for 25-30 minutes, or until the squash is tender.
3. you can Use an immersion blender to blend the soup until it become smooth. Alternatively, transfer the soup in batches to a blender and blend until smooth, then return it to the pot.
4. Add Season to the soup (salt and pepper) to taste if you desired. Serve hot, garnished with a dollop of Greek yogurt or a drizzle of coconut cream if desired.

Nutritional Information (per serving):

Calories: Approximately 150-180 kcal

Total Fat: Around 3-4 grams

Sodium: Approximately 400-500 milligrams

Total Carbohydrates: Approximately 30-35 grams

Dietary Fiber: Approximately 5-7 grams

Sugars: Approximately 6-8 grams

Protein: Around 3-4 grams

Spinach and Strawberry Salad

Serving Size: Approximately 1 cup, Prep Time: 10 minutes, Total Time: 10 minutes

Ingredients:

- 2 cups of baby spinach leaves, rinsed and patted dry
- 1 cup sliced strawberries
- 1/4 cup crumbled feta cheese or goat cheese
- 2 tablespoons sliced almonds or chopped walnuts
- Balsamic vinaigrette dressing:
- 2 tablespoons balsamic vinegar
- 1 tablespoon olive oil
- 1 teaspoon honey or maple syrup
- Salt and pepper to taste

Directions:

1. In a very big bowl, mix together the baby spinach, sliced strawberries, crumbled feta cheese, and either sliced almonds or chopped walnuts.
2. In a small bowl, whisk together the balsamic vinegar, olive oil, honey or maple syrup, salt, and pepper to make the dressing.
3. Drizzle the dressing over the salad and toss gently to coat evenly.
4. Serve the spinach and strawberry salad immediately as a refreshing and nutritious side dish or light meal.

Nutritional Information (per serving):

Calories: Approximately 120-150 kcal

Total Fat: Around 7-9 grams

Sodium: Approximately 150-200 milligrams

Total Carbohydrates: Approximately 10-12 grams

Dietary Fiber: Approximately 3-4 grams

Sugars: Approximately 6-8 grams

Protein: Around 4-5 grams

Chicken and Vegetable Rice Soup

Serving Size: Approximately 1 1/2 cups, Prep Time: 15 minutes, Cooking Time: 25 minutes, Total Time: 40 minutes

Ingredients:

- 1 tablespoon olive oil
- 1 onion, diced
- 2 carrots, peeled and diced
- 2 celery stalks, diced
- 2 cloves garlic, minced
- 6 cups low-sodium chicken broth
- 1 cup of cooked chicken breast, shredded or chopped
- 1/2 cup brown rice, uncooked
- 1 cup mixed vegetables (such as peas, corn, and green beans)
- Salt and pepper to taste
- Fresh parsley for garnish (optional)

Directions:

1. In a very big pot, warm olive oil over medium heat. Add the onion, carrots, celery, and garlic, and sauté until softened, about 5 minutes.
2. Put all the chicken broth together and boil them. Add the cooked chicken breast, brown rice, and mixed vegetables to the pot.
3. Reduce the heat to low, cover, and simmer for 20-25 minutes, or until the rice is cooked and the vegetables are tender.
4. Add Season to the soup (salt and pepper) to taste. Serve it hot, garnished with fresh parsley if you wish.

Nutritional Information (per serving):

Calories: Approximately 200-230 kcal

Total Fat: Around 4-5 grams

Sodium: Approximately 300-400 milligrams

Total Carbohydrates: Approximately 20-25 grams

Dietary Fiber: Approximately 3-4 grams

Sugars: Approximately 4-6 grams

Protein: Around 15-18 grams

Quinoa Vegetable Soup

Serving Size: Approximately 1 1/2 cups, Prep Time: 15 minutes, Cooking Time: 30 minutes, Total Time: 45 minutes

Ingredients:

- 1 tablespoon olive oil
- 1 onion, diced
- 2 carrots, peeled and diced
- 2 celery stalks, diced

- 2 cloves garlic, minced
- 4 cups low-sodium vegetable broth
- 1 can (15 ounces) diced tomatoes
- 1/2 cup quinoa, rinsed
- 1 teaspoon dried thyme
- 1/2 teaspoon dried oregano
- Salt and pepper to taste
- 2 cups chopped kale or spinach
- 1 tablespoon lemon juice
- Fresh parsley for garnish (optional)

Directions:

1. In a very big pot, warm olive oil over medium heat. Add the onion, carrots, celery, and garlic, and sauté until softened, about 5 minutes.
2. Add in the vegetable broth and bring to a boil. Add the diced tomatoes (with juices), quinoa, dried thyme, dried oregano, salt, and pepper to the pot.
3. Reduce the heat to low, cover, and simmer for 20-25 minutes, or until the quinoa is cooked and the vegetables are tender.
4. Stir in the chopped kale or spinach and lemon juice. Continue cooking for another 5 minutes, until the greens have wilted.
5. Taste and adjust seasoning as needed. Serve it hot, garnished with fresh parsley if you wish.

Nutritional Information (per serving):

Calories: Approximately 180-200 kcal

Total Fat: Around 4-5 grams

Sodium: Approximately 400-500 milligrams

Total Carbohydrates: Approximately 30-35 grams

Dietary Fiber: Approximately 5-7 grams

Sugars: Approximately 5-7 grams

Protein: Around 8-10 grams

Arugula and Beet Salad with Citrus Dressing

Serving Size: Approximately 1 cup, Prep Time: 15 minutes, Total Time: 15 minutes

Ingredients:

- 2 cups baby arugula
- 1 cup cooked beets, diced
- 1/4 cup of goat cheese or feta cheese, crumbled
- 2 tablespoons chopped walnuts or pecans

Citrus dressing:

- 2 tablespoons orange juice
- 1 tablespoon lemon juice
- 1 tablespoon extra virgin olive oil
- 1 teaspoon honey or maple syrup
- Salt and pepper to taste

Directions:

1. In a large bowl, combine the baby arugula, diced beets, crumbled goat cheese, and chopped nuts.
2. In a small bowl, whisk together the orange juice, lemon juice, olive oil, honey or maple syrup, salt, and pepper to make the dressing.
3. Drizzle the dressing over the salad and toss gently to coat evenly.
4. Serve the arugula and beet salad immediately as a refreshing and nutritious side dish or light meal.

Nutritional Information (per serving):

Calories: Approximately 150-180 kcal

Total Fat: Around 9-10 grams

Sodium: Approximately 150-200 milligrams

Total Carbohydrates: Approximately 15-20 grams

Dietary Fiber: Approximately 3-4 grams

Sugars: Approximately 8-10 grams

Protein: Around 4-5 grams

Chicken and Vegetable Salad with Balsamic Vinaigrette

Serving Size: Approximately 1 1/2 cups, Prep Time: 20 minutes, Cooking Time: 15 minutes, Total Time: 35 minutes

Ingredients:

- 1 boneless, skinless chicken breast
- 1 tablespoon olive oil
- Salt and pepper to taste
- 4 cups mixed salad greens (such as lettuce, spinach, and arugula)
- 1 cup cherry tomatoes, halved
- 1/2 cucumber, sliced
- 1/4 red onion, thinly sliced
- ¼ cup sliced almonds or chopped walnuts

Balsamic vinaigrette dressing:

- 2 tablespoons balsamic vinegar
- 1 tablespoon extra virgin olive oil
- 1 teaspoon Dijon mustard
- 1 teaspoon honey or maple syrup
- Salt and pepper to taste

Directions:

1. Preheat the oven to 400°F (200°C). Season the chicken breast with salt and pepper, and drizzle with olive oil. Place the chicken on a baking sheet and bake for 15-20 minutes, or until cooked through. Let it cool slightly, then slice or shred the chicken.

2. In a large bowl, combine the mixed salad greens, cherry tomatoes, cucumber, red onion, and sliced almonds or chopped walnuts.

3. In a small bowl, whisk together the balsamic vinegar, olive oil, Dijon mustard, honey or maple syrup, salt, and pepper to make the dressing.

4. Add the sliced or shredded chicken to the salad, drizzle with the balsamic vinaigrette dressing, and toss gently to coat evenly.

5. Serve the chicken and vegetable salad immediately as a satisfying and nutritious meal.

Nutritional Information (per serving):

Calories: Approximately 250-300 kcal

Total Fat: Around 15-18 grams

Sodium: Approximately 200-250 milligrams

Total Carbohydrates: Approximately 15-20 grams

Dietary Fiber: Approximately 4-5 grams

Sugars: Approximately 6-8 grams

Protein: Around 18-20 grams

Lentil Spinach Soup

Serving Size: Approximately 1 1/2 cups, Prep Time: 15 minutes, Cooking Time: 35 minutes, Total Time: 50 minutes

Ingredients:

- 1 cup of dried green or brown lentils, washed and drained
- 4 cups low-sodium vegetable broth
- 1 onion, diced
- 2 carrots, peeled and diced
- 2 celery stalks, diced
- 2 cloves garlic, minced

- 1 teaspoon ground cumin
- 1/2 teaspoon ground turmeric
- 1/2 teaspoon paprika
- Salt and pepper to taste
- 4 cups fresh spinach leaves
- 1 tablespoon lemon juice
- Fresh cilantro for garnish (optional)

Directions:

1. In a large pot, combine the lentils, vegetable broth, onion, carrots, celery, garlic, cumin, turmeric, paprika, salt, and pepper. Heat over medium-high heat until it boils.
2. Lower the heat to a gentle simmer, cover the pot, and let it cook for 25-30 minutes, or until the lentils and vegetables have become tender.
3. Stir in the fresh spinach leaves and lemon juice. Cook for an additional 5 minutes, until the spinach is wilted.
4. Taste and adjust seasoning as needed. Serve it hot, garnished with fresh cilantro if you wish.

Nutritional Information (per serving):

Calories: Approximately 180-200 kcal

Total Fat: Around 1-2 grams

Sodium: Approximately 400-500 milligrams

Total Carbohydrates: Approximately 30-35 grams

Dietary Fiber: Approximately 12-15 grams

Sugars: Approximately 4-6 grams

Protein: Around 10-12 grams

Quinoa Avocado Salad

Serving Size: Approximately 1 cup, Prep Time: 20 minutes, Total Time: 20 minutes

Ingredients:

- 1 cup cooked quinoa, cooled
- 1 ripe avocado, diced
- 1 cup cherry tomatoes, halved
- 1/4 cup diced red onion
- 1/4 cup chopped fresh cilantro
- 1 tablespoon lime juice
- 1 tablespoon extra virgin olive oil
- Salt and pepper to taste

Directions:

1. In a very big bowl, mix all the prepared quinoa together, chopped avocado, cherry tomatoes, red onion, and cilantro.
2. In a tiny bowl, blend the lime juice, olive oil, salt, and pepper thoroughly to create the dressing.
3. Drizzle the dressing over the salad and toss gently to coat evenly.
4. Serve the quinoa avocado salad immediately as a refreshing and nutritious side dish or light meal.

Nutritional Information (per serving):

Calories: Approximately 180-200 kcal

Total Fat: Around 10-12 grams

Sodium: Approximately 150-200 milligrams

Total Carbohydrates: Approximately 20-25 grams

Dietary Fiber: Approximately 5-7 grams

Sugars: Approximately 2-4 grams

Protein: Around 4-5 grams

Tomato Basil Soup

Serving Size: Approximately 1 1/2 cups, Prep Time: 15 minutes, Cooking Time: 30 minutes, Total Time: 45 minutes

Ingredients:

- 1 tablespoon olive oil
- 1 onion, diced
- 2 cloves garlic, minced
- 4 cups low-sodium vegetable broth
- 2 cans (14.5 ounces each) diced tomatoes
- 1/4 cup chopped fresh basil leaves
- 1 teaspoon dried oregano
- Salt and pepper to taste
- Optional: ¼ cup heavy cream or coconut milk for a creamier soup

Directions:

1. In a very big pot, warm olive oil over medium heat. Add the onion and garlic, cooking until they become soft and fragrant, typically around 3 to 4 minutes.
2. Add in the vegetable broth and bring it to a simmer. Add the diced tomatoes (with juices), fresh basil, dried oregano, salt, and pepper to the pot.
3. Simmer the soup for 20-25 minutes, stirring occasionally, to allow the flavors to meld together.
4. If desired, use an immersion blender to puree the soup until smooth. Alternatively, transfer the soup in batches to a blender and blend until smooth, then return it to the pot.
5. If using, stir in the heavy cream or coconut milk for a creamier texture. Taste and adjust seasoning as needed.
6. Serve the tomato basil soup piping hot, optionally adorned with extra fresh basil leaves if preferred.

Nutritional Information (per serving, without cream):

Calories: Approximately 100-120 kcal

Total Fat: Around 3-4 grams

Sodium: Approximately 400-500 milligrams

Total Carbohydrates: Approximately 15-20 grams

Dietary Fiber: Approximately 4-6 grams

Sugars: Approximately 8-10 grams

Protein: Around 2-3 grams

CHAPTER 4

PROTEIN-PACKED SNACKS

Spinach Egg Salad

Serving Size: 1 serving, Prep Time: 10 minutes, Cooking Time: 10 minutes, Total Time: 20 minutes

Ingredients:

- 1 cup of fresh spinach leaves, rinsed and thoroughly dried
- 1 hard-boiled egg, sliced
- 1/4 cup cherry tomatoes, halved
- 1/4 avocado, diced
- 1 tablespoon balsamic vinaigrette dressing
- Salt and pepper to taste

Directions:

1. In a medium bowl, combine the fresh spinach leaves, sliced hard-boiled egg, cherry tomatoes, and diced avocado.
2. Drizzle the balsamic vinaigrette dressing over the salad and toss gently to coat evenly.
3. Season with salt and pepper to taste.
4. Serve immediately as a protein-packed snack or light meal.

Nutritional Information (per serving):

Calories: Approximately 200 kcal

Total Fat: Around 14 grams

Sodium: Approximately 150 milligrams

Total Carbohydrates: Approximately 10 grams

Dietary Fiber: Approximately 4 grams

Sugars: Approximately 2 grams

Protein: Around 10 grams

Avocado Hummus Toast

Serving Size: 1 serving (2 slices of toast), Prep Time: 5 minutes, Cooking Time: 5 minutes, Total Time: 10 minutes

Ingredients:

- 2 slices whole grain bread, toasted
- 1/2 ripe avocado, mashed
- 1/4 cup hummus (store-bought or homemade)
- Pinch of red pepper flakes (optional)
- Fresh cilantro or parsley for garnish (optional)

Directions:

1. Evenly spread the mashed avocado onto the toasted whole-grain bread slices.
2. Top each slice with a generous dollop of hummus.
3. Sprinkle with red pepper flakes, if desired, for a bit of spice.
4. Add fresh cilantro or parsley as a garnish, if you like.
5. Serve immediately as a protein-packed snack or light meal.

Nutritional Information (per serving):

Calories: Approximately 250 kcal

Total Fat: Around 12 grams

Sodium: Approximately 300 milligrams

Total Carbohydrates: Approximately 28 grams

Dietary Fiber: Approximately 8 grams

Sugars: Approximately 2 grams

Protein: Around 10 grams

Curry Hummus

Serving Size: Approximately 1/4 cup, Prep Time: 10 minutes, Total Time: 10 minutes

Ingredients:

- 1 can (15 ounces) of chickpeas, washed and drained
- 2 tablespoons tahini
- 1 tablespoon olive oil
- 2 cloves garlic, minced
- 1 teaspoon curry powder
- 1/2 teaspoon ground cumin
- 1/4 teaspoon ground turmeric
- Juice of 1 lemon
- Salt and pepper to taste
- Water (as needed for desired consistency)

Directions:

1. In a food processor, combine the chickpeas, tahini, olive oil, minced garlic, curry powder, ground cumin, ground turmeric, and lemon juice.
2. Blend until creamy, adding water as necessary to achieve the consistency you prefer.
3. Season with salt and pepper according to your taste, and reduce the seasoning if needed.
4. Move the curry hummus to a serving dish.
5. Serve with vegetable sticks, whole grain crackers, or as a spread on sandwiches.
6. Keep any remaining portions in a sealed container in the fridge, where they can last for up to a week.

Nutritional Information (per serving):

Calories: Approximately 100 kcal

Total Fat: Around 5 grams

Sodium: Approximately 150 milligrams

Total Carbohydrates: Approximately 10 grams

Dietary Fiber: Approximately 3 grams

Sugars: Approximately 1 gram

Protein: Around 4 grams

Lemon-Herb Chicken Salad

Serving Size: 1 serving, Prep Time: 15 minutes, Cooking Time: 20 minutes, Total Time: 35 minutes

Ingredients:

- 1 boneless, skinless chicken breast
- 1 tablespoon olive oil
- Salt and pepper to taste
- 1/4 cup Greek yogurt
- 1 tablespoon fresh lemon juice
- 1 teaspoon lemon zest
- 1 tablespoon of freshly chopped herbs (like parsley, dill, or chives)
- 1/4 cup diced celery
- 2 tablespoons diced red onion
- Optional: lettuce leaves or whole grain bread for serving

Directions:

1. Preheat the oven to 375°F (190°C). Season the chicken breast with salt and pepper, and drizzle with olive oil.
2. Put the chicken on a baking sheet and bake it for 20-25 minutes, or until it's fully cooked. Let it cool slightly, then dice or shred the chicken.
3. In a mixing bowl, combine the Greek yogurt, lemon juice, lemon zest, chopped fresh herbs, diced celery, and diced red onion.
4. Add the diced or shredded chicken to the yogurt mixture and toss gently to coat evenly.

5. Serve the lemon-herb chicken salad on lettuce leaves for a low-carb option or in whole grain bread for a heartier snack.

Nutritional Information (per serving):

Calories: Approximately 250 kcal

Total Fat: Around 10 grams

Sodium: Approximately 200 milligrams

Total Carbohydrates: Approximately 4 grams

Dietary Fiber: Approximately 1 gram

Sugars: Approximately 2 grams

Protein: Around 35 grams

Avocado Tuna Boats

Serving Size: 1 serving (2 halves), Prep Time: 10 minutes, Total Time: 10 minutes

Ingredients:

- 1 ripe avocado, halved and pitted
- 1 can (5 ounces) tuna, drained
- 1 tablespoon Greek yogurt or mayonnaise
- 1 tablespoon chopped fresh cilantro or parsley
- 1 teaspoon lime juice
- Salt and pepper to taste
- Optional: cherry tomatoes or sliced cucumber for garnish

Directions:

1. In a small mixing bowl, combine the drained tuna, Greek yogurt, or mayonnaise, chopped fresh cilantro or parsley, lime juice, salt, and pepper.

2. Scoop out a little bit of avocado flesh from each avocado half to create a larger cavity for the tuna filling.

3. Fill each avocado half with the tuna mixture.

4. Garnish with cherry tomatoes or sliced cucumber, if desired.

5. Serve the avocado tuna boats immediately as a satisfying and nutritious snack.

Nutritional Information (per serving):

Calories: Approximately 250 kcal

Total Fat: Around 15 grams

Sodium: Approximately 250 milligrams

Total Carbohydrates: Approximately 10 grams

Dietary Fiber: Approximately 7 grams

Sugars: Approximately 1 gram

Protein: Around 20 grams

Smoked Salmon and Goat Cheese Toast

Serving Size: 1 serving, Prep Time: 5 minutes, Total Time: 5 minutes

Ingredients:

- 1 slice whole grain bread, toasted
- 2 ounces smoked salmon
- 1 tablespoon soft goat cheese
- 1 teaspoon capers
- Fresh dill for garnish
- Optional: lemon wedge for serving

Directions:

1. Spread the soft goat cheese evenly onto the toasted whole-grain bread slice.

2. Top with smoked salmon and sprinkle with capers.

3. Garnish with fresh dill.

4. Serve the smoked salmon and goat cheese toast immediately, with a lemon wedge on the side if desired.

Nutritional Information (per serving):

Calories: Approximately 200 kcal

Total Fat: Around 8 grams

Sodium: Approximately 600 milligrams

Total Carbohydrates: Approximately 15 grams

Dietary Fiber: Approximately 3 grams

Sugars: Approximately 2 grams

Protein: Around 15 grams

Garlic-Herb Yogurt Dip

Serving Size: 1 serving (2 tablespoons), Prep Time: 5 minutes, Total Time: 5 minutes

Ingredients:

- 1/2 cup Greek yogurt
- 1 clove garlic, minced
- 1 tablespoon of freshly diced herbs (such as parsley, dill, or chives)
- 1 teaspoon lemon juice
- Salt and pepper to taste
- Optional: vegetable sticks or whole grain crackers for serving

Directions:

1. In a small mixing bowl, combine the Greek yogurt, minced garlic, chopped fresh herbs, lemon juice, salt, and pepper.

2. Stir until well combined.

3. Taste and adjust seasoning as needed.

4. Serve the garlic-herb yogurt dip immediately with vegetable sticks or whole-grain crackers for dipping.

Nutritional Information (per serving):

Calories: Approximately 30 kcal

Total Fat: Around 0 grams

Sodium: Approximately 20 milligrams

Total Carbohydrates: Approximately 2 grams

Dietary Fiber: Approximately 0 grams

Sugars: Approximately 1 gram

Protein: Around 5 grams

Cinnamon-Spiced Apple Slices

Serving Size: 1 apple (2 servings), Prep Time: 5 minutes, Cooking Time: 5 minutes, Total Time: 10 minutes

Ingredients:

- 1 apple
- 1 teaspoon ground cinnamon
- 1 tablespoon almond butter or peanut butter
- Optional: honey or maple syrup for drizzling

Directions:

1. Remove the core from the apple and slice it thinly.

2. Sprinkle the apple slices with ground cinnamon.

3. Heat a non-stick skillet over medium heat. Place the apple slices in the skillet and cook for 2-3 minutes on each side, or until lightly softened.

4. Serve the cinnamon-spiced apple slices with almond butter or peanut butter for dipping.

5. Optionally, drizzle with honey or maple syrup for added sweetness.

Nutritional Information (per serving):

Calories: Approximately 80 kcal

Total Fat: Around 3 grams

Sodium: Approximately 0 milligrams

Total Carbohydrates: Approximately 15 grams

Dietary Fiber: Approximately 3 grams

Sugars: Approximately 10 grams

Protein: Around 1 gram

Dark Chocolate Brownie Bites

Serving Size: 1 bite (12 servings), Prep Time: 10 minutes, Cooking Time: 20 minutes, Total Time: 30 minutes

Ingredients:

-   1 cup black beans, drained and rinsed
-   1/4 cup unsweetened cocoa powder
-   1/4 cup honey or maple syrup
-   2 tablespoons almond butter or peanut butter
-   1 teaspoon vanilla extract
-   1/4 teaspoon baking powder
-   1/4 cup dark chocolate chips
-   Optional: chopped nuts for topping

Directions:

1. Preheat the oven to 350°F (175°C). Grease a mini muffin tin or line with mini muffin liners.
2. In a food processor, combine the black beans, cocoa powder, honey or maple syrup, almond butter or peanut butter, vanilla extract, and baking powder. Blend until smooth.
3. Stir in the dark chocolate chips.
4. Spoon the batter into the prepared mini muffin tin, filling each cavity about two-thirds full.
5. Bake for 15-20 minutes, or until set.
6. Allow the brownie bites to cool in the muffin tin for 5 minutes before transferring them to a wire rack to cool down completely.
7. Optionally, top with chopped nuts before serving.

Nutritional Information (per serving):

Calories: Approximately 70 kcal

Total Fat: Around 3 grams

Sodium: Approximately 30 milligrams

Total Carbohydrates: Approximately 11 grams

Dietary Fiber: Approximately 2 grams

Sugars: Approximately 6 grams

Protein: Around 2 grams

Vegan Banana-Walnut Ice Cream

Serving Size: 1/2 cup (4 servings), Prep Time: 5 minutes, Freezing Time: 4 hours

Total Time: 4 hours 5 minutes

Ingredients:

- 2 ripe bananas, sliced and frozen
- 1/4 cup coconut milk or almond milk

- 1/4 cup chopped walnuts
- 1 teaspoon vanilla extract
- Optional: Maple syrup or honey for added sweetness

Directions:

1. In a blender or food processor, combine the frozen banana slices, coconut milk or almond milk, chopped walnuts, and vanilla extract.
2. Blend until the mixture is smooth and creamy, occasionally scraping down the sides of the blender or food processor.
3. Taste the mixture and add maple syrup or honey if desired for added sweetness.
4. Move the mixture to a container safe for freezing and freeze it for at least 4 hours, or until it becomes firm.
5. Let the vegan banana-walnut ice cream sit at room temperature for a few minutes before scooping and serving.

Nutritional Information (per serving):

Calories: Approximately 120 kcal

Total Fat: Around 6 grams

Sodium: Approximately 5 milligrams

Total Carbohydrates: Approximately 18 grams

Dietary Fiber: Approximately 3 grams

Sugars: Approximately 10 grams

Protein: Around 2 grams

Miso-Tahini Dip

Serving Size: 2 tablespoons (8 servings), Prep Time: 5 minutes. Total Time: 5 minutes

Ingredients:

- 1/4 cup tahini
- 1 tablespoon white miso paste
- 1 tablespoon lemon juice
- 1 clove garlic, minced
- 2 tablespoons water
- Optional: sesame seeds for garnish

Directions:

1. In a small bowl, whisk together the tahini, white miso paste, lemon juice, minced garlic, and water until smooth.
2. If the dip is too thick, add more water, 1 teaspoon at a time, until the desired consistency is reached.
3. Add sesame seeds on top before serving, if you like.
4. Serve the miso-tahini dip with vegetable sticks, whole grain crackers, or as a spread on sandwiches.

Nutritional Information (per serving):

Calories: Approximately 50 kcal

Total Fat: Around 4 grams

Sodium: Approximately 90 milligrams

Total Carbohydrates: Approximately 3 grams

Dietary Fiber: Approximately 1 gram

Sugars: Approximately 0 grams

Protein: Around 2 grams

CHAPTER 5

STRENGTHENING MEALS

Spaghetti with Mushroom Bolognese

Serving Size: 1 serving, Prep Time: 10 minutes, Cooking Time: 30 minutes, Total Time: 40 minutes

Ingredients:

- 2 cups whole wheat or gluten-free spaghetti
- 2 cups cremini mushrooms, finely chopped
- 1 onion, diced
- 2 cloves garlic, minced
- 1 carrot, grated
- 1 celery stalk, diced
- 1 can (14.5 ounces) diced tomatoes
- 1 tablespoon tomato paste
- 1 teaspoon dried oregano
- 1 teaspoon dried basil
- Salt and pepper to taste
- Fresh parsley for garnish
- Grated Parmesan cheese (optional)

Directions:

1. Cook the spaghetti according to package instructions until al dente. Drain and set aside.
2. In a large skillet, heat olive oil over medium heat. Put in the chopped onion and minced garlic, cooking until they become soft and fragrant, typically around 3 to 4 minutes.
3. Add the chopped mushrooms, grated carrot, and diced celery to the skillet. Cook, stirring occasionally, until the vegetables are tender and the mushrooms release their juices, about 5-7 minutes.

 P a g e

4. Stir in the diced tomatoes, tomato paste, dried oregano, dried basil, salt, and pepper. Let the sauce simmer for 10-15 minutes, allowing the flavors to blend and the sauce to become thicker. Serve the mushroom bolognese sauce over cooked spaghetti, garnished with fresh parsley and grated Parmesan cheese if desired.

Nutritional Information (per serving):

Calories: Approximately 350 kcal

Total Fat: Around 2 grams

Sodium: Approximately 400 milligrams

Total Carbohydrates: Approximately 70 grams

Dietary Fiber: Approximately 10 grams

Sugars: Approximately 10 grams

Protein: Around 15 grams

Mushroom Burgers

Serving Size: 1 burger, Prep Time: 15 minutes, Cooking Time: 15 minutes, Total Time: 30 minutes

Ingredients:

-   2 cups of mushrooms (like portobello or cremini), finely diced
-   1 onion, finely chopped
-   2 cloves garlic, minced
-   1/2 cup rolled oats
-   1/4 cup breadcrumbs (whole wheat or gluten-free)
-   1 tablespoon soy sauce or tamari
-   1 teaspoon dried thyme
-   Salt and pepper to taste
-   Whole grain burger buns
-   Lettuce, tomato slices, and avocado slices to use as garnish.

Directions:

1. In a large skillet, heat olive oil over medium heat. Add the chopped mushrooms, onion, and minced garlic. Sauté until the mushrooms are tender and the onions are translucent about 5-7 minutes.

2. Move the cooked mushroom mixture to a food processor. Add the rolled oats, breadcrumbs, soy sauce or tamari, dried thyme, salt, and pepper. Pulse until well combined and the mixture holds together.

3. Shape the mushroom mixture into burger patties.

4. In the same skillet, heat a little more olive oil over medium heat. Cook the mushroom burgers for 3-4 minutes per side, or until they turn golden brown and are heated thoroughly.

5. Serve the mushroom burgers on whole grain burger buns, garnished with lettuce, tomato slices, and avocado slices.

Nutritional Information (per serving):

Calories: Approximately 250 kcal

Total Fat: Around 5 grams

Sodium: Approximately 400 milligrams

Total Carbohydrates: Approximately 45 grams

Dietary Fiber: Approximately 8 grams

Sugars: Approximately 5 grams

Protein: Around 10 grams

Turkey-Stuffed Zucchini

Serving Size: 1 zucchini boat, Prep Time: 15 minutes, Cooking Time: 30 minutes, Total Time: 45 minutes

Ingredients:

- 2 medium zucchini
- 1/2 pound lean ground turkey
- 1 onion, diced

- 1 bell pepper, diced

- 2 cloves garlic, minced

- 1 teaspoon dried oregano

- 1 teaspoon dried basil

- 1 can (14.5 ounces) diced tomatoes

- Salt and pepper to taste

- Grated Parmesan cheese for topping (optional)

- Fresh basil for garnish

Directions:

1. Preheat the oven to 375°F (190°C). Cut the zucchini in half lengthwise and scoop out the seeds to create zucchini boats.

2. In a large skillet, cook the ground turkey over medium heat until browned and cooked through, breaking it apart with a spoon as it cooks. Drain any excess fat.

3. Add the diced onion, bell pepper, and minced garlic to the skillet with the cooked turkey. Cook until the vegetables become tender, approximately 5-7 minutes.

4. Stir in the dried oregano, dried basil, diced tomatoes (with juices), salt, and pepper. Simmer the mixture for 5-10 minutes to allow the flavors to meld together.

5. Place the zucchini boats in a baking dish. Fill each boat with the turkey and vegetable mixture.

6. Bake in the preheated oven for 20-25 minutes, or until the zucchini is tender.

7. Optionally, sprinkle the stuffed zucchini boats with grated Parmesan cheese before serving. Garnish with fresh basil.

Nutritional Information (per serving):

Calories: Approximately 200 kcal

Total Fat: Around 5 grams

Sodium: Approximately 400 milligrams

Total Carbohydrates: Approximately 15 grams

Dietary Fiber: Approximately 5 grams

Sugars: Approximately 8 grams

Protein: Around 20 grams

Moroccan-Spiced Zucchini

Serving Size: 1 serving, Prep Time: 10 minutes, Cooking Time: 20 minutes, Total Time: 30 minutes

Ingredients:

- 2 medium zucchini, sliced into rounds
- 1 tablespoon olive oil
- 1 teaspoon ground cumin
- 1/2 teaspoon ground coriander
- 1/2 teaspoon ground cinnamon
- 1/4 teaspoon ground ginger
- 1/4 teaspoon ground turmeric
- Salt and pepper to taste
- Fresh cilantro for garnish

Directions:

1. In a large skillet, heat olive oil over medium heat. Add the sliced zucchini rounds to the skillet.
2. Sprinkle the ground cumin, ground coriander, ground cinnamon, ground ginger, ground turmeric, salt, and pepper over the zucchini rounds. Toss to coat evenly.
3. Cook the zucchini rounds for 15-20 minutes, stirring occasionally, until tender and golden brown.
4. Serve the Moroccan-spiced zucchini hot, garnished with fresh cilantro.

Nutritional Information (per serving):

Calories: Approximately 80 kcal

Total Fat: Around 5 grams

Sodium: Approximately 300 milligrams

Total Carbohydrates: Approximately 8 grams

Dietary Fiber: Approximately 3 grams

Sugars: Approximately 5 grams

Protein: Around 3 grams

Walnut Chicken and Pomegranate

Serving Size: 1 serving, Prep Time: 10 minutes, Cooking Time: 20 minutes, Total Time: 30 minutes

Ingredients:

- 1 boneless, skinless chicken breast
- 1/4 cup walnuts, chopped
- 1/4 cup pomegranate arils
- 1 tablespoon olive oil
- 1 tablespoon honey
- 1 teaspoon Dijon mustard
- Salt and pepper to taste
- Fresh parsley for garnish

Directions:

1. Season the chicken breast with salt and pepper. Warm olive oil in a skillet on medium heat.
2. Cook the chicken breast for 6-8 minutes on each side, or until cooked through.
3. In a small bowl, combine honey and Dijon mustard, whisking them together. After the chicken is cooked, take it out of the skillet and allow it to rest for a few minutes. Slice the chicken.
4. In the same skillet, add the chopped walnuts and toast them for 2-3 minutes, stirring frequently.
5. Serve the sliced chicken topped with toasted walnuts, and pomegranate arils, and drizzle with the honey-Dijon mixture. Garnish with fresh parsley.

Nutritional Information (per serving):

Calories: Approximately 300 kcal

Total Fat: Around 15 grams

Sodium: Approximately 150 milligrams

Total Carbohydrates: Approximately 15 grams

Dietary Fiber: Approximately 2 grams

Sugars: Approximately 12 grams

Protein: Around 25 grams

Turkey and Bean Chili

Serving Size: 1 serving, Prep Time: 15 minutes, Cooking Time: 30 minutes, Total Time: 45 minutes

Ingredients:

- 1 pound lean ground turkey
- 1 onion, diced
- 2 cloves garlic, minced
- 1 bell pepper, diced
- 1 can (14.5 ounces) diced tomatoes
- 1 can (15 ounces) of kidney beans, washed and drained
- 1 can (15 ounces)of black beans, washed and drained
- 2 tablespoons chili powder
- 1 teaspoon ground cumin
- Salt and pepper to taste
- Optional toppings: chopped cilantro, shredded cheese, Greek yogurt

Directions:

1. In a large pot, cook the ground turkey on medium heat until it's browned.
2. Add the diced onion, minced garlic, and diced bell pepper to the pot. Cook until the vegetables are soft, approximately 5 minutes.
3. Stir in the diced tomatoes, kidney beans, black beans, chili powder, and ground cumin.
4. Bring the chili to a simmer and cook for 20-25 minutes, stirring occasionally.
5. Season with salt and pepper to taste.

6. Serve the turkey and bean chili hot, topped with optional toppings like chopped cilantro, shredded cheese, or a dollop of Greek yogurt.

Nutritional Information (per serving):

Calories: Approximately 350 kcal

Total Fat: Around 8 grams

Sodium: Approximately 600 milligrams

Total Carbohydrates: Approximately 35 grams

Dietary Fiber: Approximately 10 grams

Sugars: Approximately 8 grams

Protein: Around 30 grams

Curried Chicken and Chickpeas

Serving Size: 1 serving, Prep Time: 10 minutes, Cooking Time: 20 minutes, Total Time: 30 minutes

Ingredients:

-   1 boneless, skinless chicken breast, diced
-   1 can (15 ounces) of chickpeas, washed and drained
-   1 onion, diced
-   2 cloves garlic, minced
-   1 tablespoon curry powder
-   1/2 teaspoon ground turmeric
-   1/4 teaspoon ground cayenne pepper (optional)
-   1 can (14.5 ounces) diced tomatoes
-   1/2 cup coconut milk
-   Salt and pepper to taste
-   Fresh cilantro for garnish

Directions:

1. In a large skillet, heat olive oil over medium heat. Include the diced chicken breast and cook until it becomes golden brown and fully cooked. Then, add the diced onion and minced garlic to the skillet. Cook until onion is translucent, about 5 minutes.
2. Stir in the curry powder, ground turmeric, and ground cayenne pepper (if using), and cook for 1 minute until fragrant.
3. Add the drained and rinsed chickpeas, diced tomatoes, and coconut milk to the skillet. Stir to combine.
4. Bring the mixture to a simmer and let it cook for 10-15 minutes, occasionally stirring.
5. Season with salt and pepper to taste.
6. Serve the curried chicken and chickpeas hot, garnished with fresh cilantro.

Nutritional Information (per serving):

Calories: Approximately 350 kcal

Total Fat: Around 12 grams

Sodium: Approximately 500 milligrams

Total Carbohydrates: Approximately 30 grams

Dietary Fiber: Approximately 8 grams

Sugars: Approximately 6 grams

Protein: Around 30 grams

Turkey Taco Salad

Serving Size: 1 serving, Prep Time: 15 minutes, Cooking Time: 15 minutes, Total Time: 30 minutes

Ingredients:

- 1 pound lean ground turkey
- 1 tablespoon olive oil
- 1 packet taco seasoning mix

- 1 head romaine lettuce, chopped
- 1 cup cherry tomatoes, halved
- 1/2 cup black beans, drained and rinsed
- 1/2 cup corn kernels (fresh or frozen)
- 1 avocado, diced
- 1/4 cup shredded cheese
- Salsa and Greek yogurt for serving

Directions:

1. In a large skillet, heat olive oil over medium heat. Add the ground turkey and cook until browned, breaking it apart with a spoon as it cooks.
2. Stir in the taco seasoning mix and cook according to package instructions.
3. In a large bowl, combine the chopped romaine lettuce, halved cherry tomatoes, black beans, corn kernels, diced avocado, and shredded cheese.
4. Add the cooked turkey mixture to the bowl and toss to combine.
5. Serve the turkey taco salad with salsa and Greek yogurt on the side.

Nutritional Information (per serving):

Calories: Approximately 400 kcal

Total Fat: Around 20 grams

Sodium: Approximately 800 milligrams

Total Carbohydrates: Approximately 25 grams

Dietary Fiber: Approximately 8 grams

Sugars: Approximately 5 grams

Protein: Around 30 grams

CHAPTER 6

HEALTHY BEVERAGES AND JUICES

Ginger-Licious Green Smoothie

(Serving size: 1 glass), Prep Time: 5 minutes

Ingredients:

- 1 cup unsweetened plant-based milk (almond milk, soy milk, etc.)
- 1 handful (about 1 cup) baby spinach or kale
- ½ banana, frozen or fresh
- 1-inch fresh ginger, peeled and chopped
- ¼ cup pineapple chunks (fresh or frozen)
- ½ teaspoon ground turmeric (optional)

Directions:

1. put all the ingredients in a blender and blend until they reach a smooth and creamy consistency.
2. If desired, add a little more plant-based milk for a thinner consistency.
3. Pour into a glass and enjoy!

Nutritional Information (per 1 glass):

Calories: 200

Fat: 3g

Saturated Fat: 1g (depending on plant-based milk used)

Carbohydrates: 35g

Fiber: 4g

Sugar: (natural sugars from fruits)

Protein: 2g (depending on plant-based milk used)

Berry-licious Antioxidant Boost

(Serving size: 1 glass), Prep Time: 5 minutes

Ingredients:

- 1 cup unsweetened pomegranate juice
- 1 cup of assorted frozen berries, including blueberries, raspberries, and strawberries.
- ½ cup sparkling water (optional, for a fizzy touch)
- ¼ cup fresh mint leaves

Directions:

1. Add the pomegranate juice, frozen berries, and mint leaves to a blender. Blend until smooth.
2. If using sparkling water, slowly add it to the blender and pulse a few times to incorporate without creating too much fizz.
3. Pour into a glass and enjoy!

Nutritional Information (per 1 glass):

Calories: 150

Fat: 0g

Saturated Fat: 0g

Carbohydrates: 30g

Fiber: 3g

Sugar: (natural sugars from fruits)

Protein: 1g (trace amounts)

Turmeric Tea with Honey

(Serving size: 1 cup), Prep Time: 5 minutes

Ingredients:

- 1 cup water
- 1 inch fresh turmeric root, peeled and grated (or 1 teaspoon ground turmeric)
- 1-inch fresh ginger root, peeled and sliced (optional)
- 1 black tea bag (optional)
- 1 tablespoon of honey (or adjust to taste with maple syrup).
- Lemon wedge (optional)

Directions:

1. In a small saucepan, combine the water, turmeric, and ginger (if using).
2. Bring the mixture to a boil, then lower the heat and let it simmer for 5 to 10 minutes.
3. If using a black tea bag, add it during the last few minutes of simmering.
4. Take the tea off the heat and pour it through a strainer into a mug.
5. Stir in honey (or maple syrup) to taste.
6. Add a lemon wedge for an extra touch of flavor (optional).

Nutritional Information (per 1 cup, with honey):

Calories: 60

Fat: 0g

Saturated Fat: 0g

Carbohydrates: 15g

Fiber: 0g

Sugar: (natural sugars from honey)

Protein: 0g

Tropical Paradise Smoothie

(Serving size: 1 glass), Prep Time: 5 minutes

Ingredients:

- 1 cup unsweetened plant-based milk (coconut milk, almond milk, etc.)
- ½ cup frozen mango chunks
- ¼ cup chopped pineapple (fresh or frozen)
- ¼ avocado, peeled and pitted
- 1 tablespoon ground flaxseed (optional, for added fiber and omega-3s)
- Pinch of ground cinnamon

Directions:

1. Put all the ingredients in a blender and blend until they are smooth and creamy.
2. If desired, add a little more plant-based milk for a thinner consistency.
3. Pour into a glass and enjoy!

Nutritional Information (per 1 glass):

Calories: 250

Fat: 12g (mostly healthy fats from avocado and coconut milk)

Saturated Fat: 4g (depending on plant-based milk used)

Carbohydrates: 30g

Fiber: 4g (depending on added flaxseed)

Sugar: (natural sugars from fruits)

Protein: 2g (depending on plant-based milk used)

Spicy Carrot & Beet Detox Juice

(Serving size: 1 glass), Prep Time: 5 minutes (requires a juicer)

Ingredients:

- 1 large carrot, peeled and chopped
- 1 medium beet, peeled and chopped
- 1 medium apple, cored and chopped
- 1-inch fresh ginger root, peeled and chopped
- ¼ inch fresh jalapeño pepper, seeded and chopped (optional, for a spicy kick)
- ½ lemon, juiced

Directions:

1. Wash and prepare all ingredients.
2. Feed the ingredients one by one through your juicer.
3. If the juice is too strong for your taste, you can dilute it with a splash of water or unsweetened green tea.
4. Pour into a glass and enjoy!

Nutritional Information (per 1 glass):

Calories: 100

Fat: 0g

Saturated Fat: 0g

Carbohydrates: 25g

Fiber: 3g (depending on juicer efficiency)

Sugar: (natural sugars from fruits)

Protein: 1g (trace amounts)

Hydrating Herbal Tea Blend

(Serving size: 1 mug), Prep Time: 5 minutes

Ingredients:

- 1 cup hot water
- 1 tablespoon dried peppermint leaves
- 1 tablespoon dried chamomile flowers
- 1 teaspoon dried hibiscus flowers (optional, for a tart flavor)
- Honey or maple syrup to taste (optional)
- Lemon wedge (optional)

Directions:

1. Heat water to boiling point.
2. Pour hot water into a mug.
3. Add dried peppermint leaves, chamomile flowers, and hibiscus flowers (if using).
4. Let the tea steep for 5-10 minutes, covered.
5. Strain the tea into a mug.
6. You may optionally add honey or maple syrup according to your taste preferences.
7. Squeeze in a lemon wedge for an extra touch of flavor (optional).

Nutritional Information (per 1 mug, without honey):

Calories: 0

Fat: 0g

Saturated Fat: 0g

Carbohydrates: 0g

Fiber: 0g

Sugar: 0g (trace amounts from hibiscus flowers if used)

Protein: 0g

Spiced Apple & Pear Cooler

(Serving size: 1 glass), Prep Time: 5 minutes

Ingredients:

- 1 cup unsweetened apple juice
- ½ cup chopped pear
- 1 cinnamon stick
- 3 cloves
- Pinch of ground ginger
- ½ teaspoon lemon juice (optional)
- Pinch of ground nutmeg (optional)

Directions:

1. In a small saucepan, combine the apple juice, chopped pear, cinnamon stick, cloves, and ginger.
2. Heat the mixture over medium heat until simmering.
3. Reduce heat and simmer for 5-7 minutes, or until the pear pieces are softened.
4. Remove the saucepan from the heat. Strain the mixture into a mug or glass, discarding the solids.
5. Stir in lemon juice and nutmeg (optional) to taste.
6. Serve warm and enjoy!

Nutritional Information (per 1 glass):

Calories: 150

Fat: 0g

Saturated Fat: 0g

Carbohydrates: 35g

Fiber: 2g (depending on pear variety)

Sugar: (natural sugars from apple juice and pear)

Protein: 0g (trace amounts)

Watermelon & Mint Refresher

(Serving size: 1 glass), Prep Time: 5 minutes

Ingredients:

- 2 cups seedless watermelon chunks, frozen
- ½ cup crushed ice
- 1 tablespoon chopped fresh mint leaves
- ¼ cup sparkling water (optional)
- Squeeze of lime juice (optional)

Directions:

1. In a blender, combine the frozen watermelon chunks and crushed ice.
2. Blend until smooth and slushy.
3. Stir in the chopped mint leaves.
4. If desired, add a splash of sparkling water for a fizzy touch.
5. Squeeze in a touch of lime juice for an extra flavor dimension (optional).
6. Pour into a glass and enjoy!

Nutritional Information (per 1 glass):

Calories: 80

Fat: 0g

Saturated Fat: 0g

Carbohydrates: 20g

Fiber: 1g (depending on watermelon variety)

Sugar: (natural sugars from watermelon)

Protein: 1g (trace amounts)

Green Power Veggie Juice

(Serving size: 1 glass), Prep Time: 5 minutes (requires a juicer)

Ingredients:

- 2 large kale leaves
- 1 cucumber, peeled and chopped
- 1 celery stalk, chopped
- 1 apple, cored and chopped (optional, for sweetness)
- ½ lemon, juiced

Directions:

1. Wash and prepare all ingredients.
2. Feed the ingredients one by one through your juicer.
3. If the juice is too strong for your taste, you can dilute it with a splash of water or unsweetened green tea.
4. Pour into a glass and enjoy!

Nutritional Information (per 1 glass):

Calories: 100

Fat: 0g

Saturated Fat: 0g

Carbohydrates: 20g

Fiber: 2g (depending on juicer efficiency)

Sugar: (natural sugars from fruits and vegetables)

Protein: 2g (trace amounts)

CHAPTER 7

BROTH, DRESSINGS AND SAUCES

Healthy Homemade Mayonnaise

Serving Size: 1 tablespoon, Prep Time: 5 minutes, Total Time: 5 minutes

Ingredients:

- 1 egg yolk
- 1 teaspoon Dijon mustard
- 1 tablespoon lemon juice
- 1/2 cup of either avocado oil or a light variety of olive oil
- Salt and pepper to taste

Directions:

1. In a small bowl, whisk together the egg yolk, Dijon mustard, and lemon juice until well combined.
2. Slowly drizzle in the avocado oil or light olive oil while whisking continuously until the mixture emulsifies and thickens.
3. Season with salt and pepper to taste.
4. Store the homemade mayonnaise in an airtight container in the refrigerator for up to one week.

Nutritional Information (per serving):

Calories: Approximately 100 kcal

Total Fat: Around 11 grams

Sodium: Approximately 10 milligrams

Total Carbohydrates: Approximately 0 grams

Protein: Around 0 grams

Fresh Salsa

Serving Size: 1/4 cup, Prep Time: 10 minutes, Total Time: 10 minutes

Ingredients:

- 2 tomatoes, diced
- 1/2 onion, finely chopped
- 1 jalapeño pepper, seeded and finely chopped
- 1/4 cup chopped fresh cilantro
- 1 tablespoon lime juice
- Salt and pepper to taste

Directions:

1. In a bowl, combine the diced tomatoes, chopped onion, chopped jalapeño pepper, chopped fresh cilantro, and lime juice.
2. Season with salt and pepper to taste.
3. Mix well to combine.
4. Serve the fresh salsa immediately or refrigerate for 30 minutes to allow the flavors to meld together.

Nutritional Information (per serving):

Calories: Approximately 15 kcal

Total Fat: Around 0 grams

Sodium: Approximately 5 milligrams

Total Carbohydrates: Approximately 3 grams

Dietary Fiber: Approximately 1 gram

Sugars: Approximately 2 grams

Protein: Around 0 grams

Herbal Citrus Marinade

Serving Size: 2 tablespoons, Prep Time: 10 minutes, Total Time: 10 minutes

Ingredients:

- 1/4 cup fresh orange juice
- 2 tablespoons lemon juice
- 2 tablespoons lime juice
- 2 cloves garlic, minced
- 2 tablespoons of freshly chopped herbs, like parsley, thyme, or rosemary
- 2 tablespoons olive oil
- Salt and pepper to taste

Directions:

1. In a bowl, whisk together the fresh orange juice, lemon juice, lime juice, minced garlic, chopped fresh herbs, and olive oil.
2. Season with salt and pepper to taste.
3. Use the herbal citrus marinade to marinate chicken, fish, tofu, or vegetables for at least 30 minutes before grilling or baking.

Nutritional Information (per serving):

Calories: Approximately 50 kcal

Total Fat: Around 5 grams

Sodium: Approximately 0 milligrams

Total Carbohydrates: Approximately 2 grams

Dietary Fiber: Approximately 0 grams

Sugars: Approximately 1 gram

Protein: Around 0 grams

Moroccan-Inspired Sauce

Serving Size: 2 tablespoons, Prep Time: 10 minutes, Cooking Time: 10 minutes, Total Time: 20 minutes

Ingredients:

- 1 tablespoon olive oil
- 1 onion, finely chopped
- 2 cloves garlic, minced
- 1 teaspoon ground cumin
- 1 teaspoon ground coriander
- 1/2 teaspoon ground cinnamon
- 1/4 teaspoon ground ginger
- 1/4 teaspoon ground paprika
- 1 can (14.5 ounces) diced tomatoes
- 2 tablespoons tomato paste
- 1/4 cup chopped fresh cilantro
- Salt and pepper to taste

Directions:

1. Heat the olive oil in a skillet over medium heat. Then, add the chopped onion and minced garlic, cooking until they become soft and aromatic, typically around 3 to 4 minutes.
2. Stir in the ground cumin, ground coriander, ground cinnamon, ground ginger, and ground paprika. Cook for 1 minute until spices are toasted and aromatic.
3. Put the diced tomatoes and tomato paste into the skillet. Let it simmer for 5 to 7 minutes, stirring occasionally, until the sauce thickens.
4. Stir in the chopped fresh cilantro. Season with salt and pepper to taste.
5. Serve the Moroccan-inspired sauce over grilled chicken, fish, tofu, or vegetables.

Nutritional Information (per serving):

Calories: Approximately 30 kcal

Total Fat: Around 2 grams

Sodium: Approximately 100 milligrams

Total Carbohydrates: Approximately 3 grams

Dietary Fiber: Approximately 1 gram

Sugars: Approximately 2 grams

Protein: Around 1 gram

Lemon-Garlic Dressing

Serving Size: 2 tablespoons, Prep Time: 5 minutes, Total Time: 5 minutes

Ingredients:

- 1/4 cup fresh lemon juice
- 2 cloves garlic, minced
- 1/4 cup extra virgin olive oil
- 1 teaspoon Dijon mustard
- 1 teaspoon honey or maple syrup (optional)
- Salt and pepper to taste

Directions:

1. In a small bowl, whisk together the Dijon mustard, honey or maple syrup, and apple cider vinegar until well combined.
2. Season with salt and pepper to taste.
3. Use the lemon-garlic dressing to drizzle over salads, grilled vegetables, or roasted chicken.

Nutritional Information (per serving):

Calories: Approximately 70 kcal

Total Fat: Around 7 grams

Sodium: Approximately 20 milligrams

Total Carbohydrates: Approximately 2 grams

Protein: Around 0 grams

Honey Mustard Dressing

Serving Size: 2 tablespoons, Prep Time: 5 minutes, Total Time: 5 minutes

Ingredients:

- 2 tablespoons Dijon mustard
- 1 tablespoon honey or maple syrup
- 2 tablespoons apple cider vinegar
- 1/4 cup extra virgin olive oil
- Salt and pepper to taste

Directions:

1. In a small bowl, blend the Dijon mustard, honey or maple syrup, and apple cider vinegar together until thoroughly mixed.
2. Gradually pour the extra virgin olive oil into the mixture while whisking constantly until the dressing becomes emulsified and thickens.
3. Season with salt and pepper to taste.
4. Use the honey mustard dressing to toss with mixed greens, roasted vegetables, or grilled chicken.

Nutritional Information (per serving):

Calories: Approximately 90 kcal

Total Fat: Around 9 grams

Sodium: Approximately 80 milligrams

Total Carbohydrates: Approximately 3 grams

Protein: Around 0 grams

Creamy Turmeric Dressing

Serving Size: 2 tablespoons, Prep Time: 5 minutes, Total Time: 5 minutes

Ingredients:

- 1/4 cup plain Greek yogurt
- 1 tablespoon extra virgin olive oil
- 1 tablespoon lemon juice
- 1 teaspoon ground turmeric
- 1 teaspoon honey or maple syrup
- Salt and pepper to taste

Directions:

1. combine the Dijon mustard, in a small bowl, honey or maple syrup, and apple cider vinegar until well incorporated.
2. Season with salt and pepper to taste.
3. Use the creamy turmeric dressing to drizzle over salads, grain bowls, or roasted vegetables.

Nutritional Information (per serving):

Calories: Approximately 60 kcal

Total Fat: Around 5 grams

Sodium: Approximately 15 milligrams

Total Carbohydrates: Approximately 3 grams

Protein: Around 2 grams

Basil-Spinach Pesto

Serving Size: 2 tablespoons, Prep Time: 10 minutes, Total Time: 10 minutes

Ingredients:

- 2 cups fresh basil leaves

- 1 cup fresh spinach leaves
- 1/4 cup walnuts or pine nuts
- 2 cloves garlic
- 1/4 cup extra virgin olive oil
- 1/4 cup grated Parmesan cheese
- Salt and pepper to taste

Directions:

1. In a food processor, combine the fresh basil leaves, fresh spinach leaves, walnuts or pine nuts, and garlic. Pulse until coarsely chopped.
2. With the food processor running, slowly drizzle in the extra virgin olive oil until the pesto reaches your desired consistency.
3. Add the grated Parmesan cheese and pulse a few more times to combine.
4. Season with salt and pepper to taste.
5. Use the basil-spinach pesto as a spread on sandwiches, a topping for grilled chicken or fish, or a sauce for pasta dishes.

Nutritional Information (per serving):

Calories: Approximately 80 kcal

Total Fat: Around 8 grams

Sodium: Approximately 50 milligrams

Total Carbohydrates: Approximately 2 grams

Protein: Around 2 grams

CONCLUSION

The recipes on these pages provide a starting point. Feel free to explore, personalize, and tailor them to your taste and dietary requirements. Don't be afraid to ask your healthcare staff for advice on incorporating these foods into your unique treatment plan.

Throughout your journey, remember the joy of fueling your body with nutritious ingredients. Savor the flavors, try new things, and enjoy the social aspects of sharing meals with loved ones. Prioritizing good nutrition does more than simply nourish your body; it also allows you to take an active role in your health and regain control during this difficult period.

Throughout your journey, remember the joy of fueling your body with nutritious ingredients. Savor the flavors, try new things, and enjoy the social aspects of sharing meals with loved ones. Prioritizing good nutrition does more than simply nourish your body; it also allows you to take an active role in your health and regain control during this difficult period.

Remember: you are not alone. The cancer community supports you, and this cookbook exemplifies the power and perseverance that each individual fighting cancer possesses. We wish you a speedy recovery, tasty meals, and a restored feeling of hope for the future.

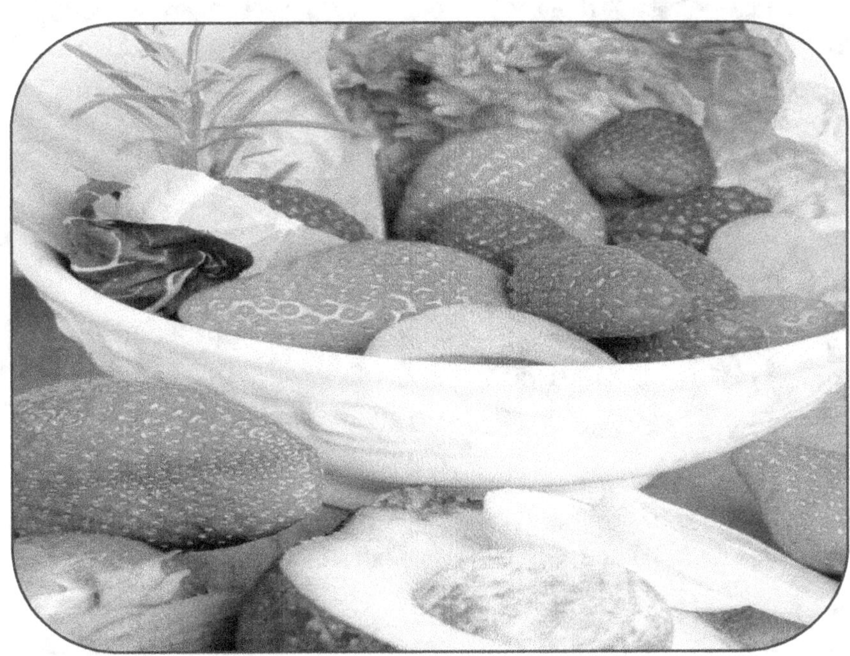

ACKNOWLEDGMENT

The creation of this cookbook would not have been possible without the invaluable contributions of many people. First and foremost, I would like to express my deepest gratitude to the cancer patients, survivors, and caregivers who have shared their stories and experiences with me. Your courage and resilience in the face of adversity have been a constant source of inspiration throughout this project.

A heartfelt thank you goes out to the dedicated team of registered dietitians and medical specialists who have contributed their expertise to ensure the correctness and nutritional soundness of the recipes shown on these pages. Their advice has been invaluable in developing a resource that is both delicious and supportive for persons undergoing cancer treatment and recovery.

Finally, I want to express my deepest appreciation to my family and friends for their unwavering love and encouragement throughout this journey. The support you've given has been incredibly meaningful to me. And also this is me saying Thank you for Buying this book.

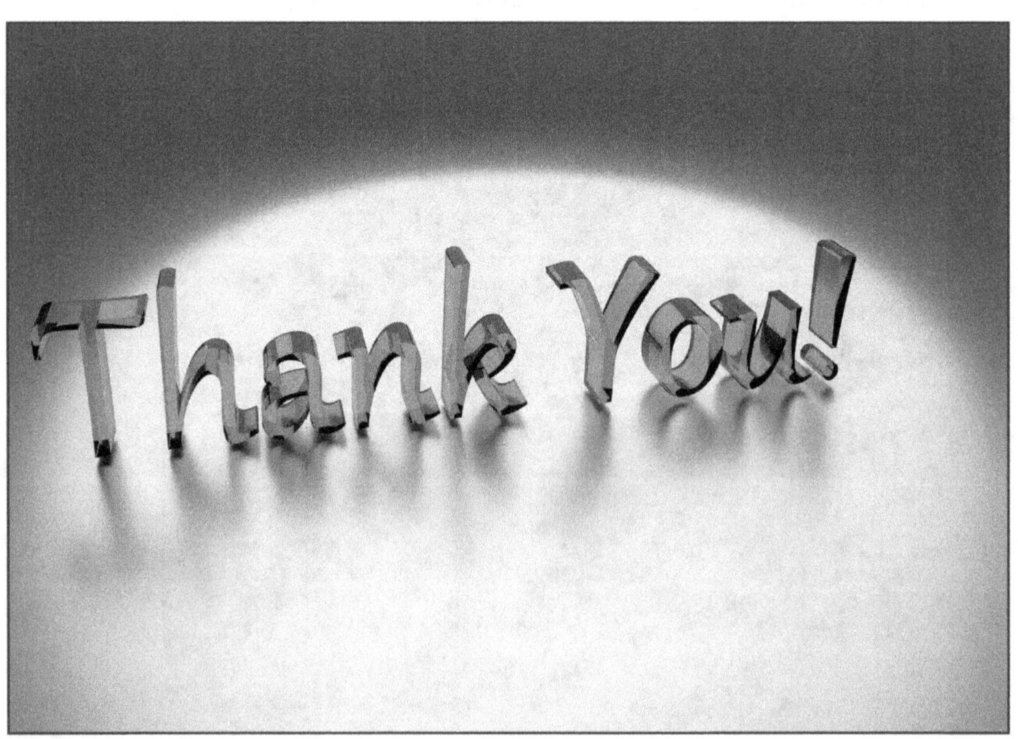